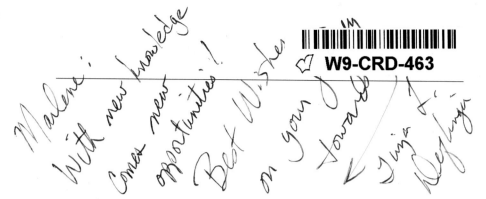

Better Breast Health — *for Life!*™

Provided by: the Breast Health Education Group

Tirza Derflinger, Founder, CTT

Deborah Breakell, NP

Carrie Louise Daenell, ND

Carol Dalton, NP

John R.M. Day, MD

Lisa High, MS, RD

Kelly McAleese, MD

Library of Congress Control Number: 2005908504
ISBN-13: 978-0-9772568-0-8
ISBN-10: 0-9772568-0-4

Published in Louisville, Colorado and printed in the U.S. This publication is available at special discounts for bulk purchases by corporations, institutions, and other organizations. For more information, or to schedule a breast health seminar or workshop at your location, contact the Breast Health Education Group at 866-492-2174 or info@BetterBreastHealthforLife.com.

Cover design and marketing support by Orbit Design, www.orbit-design.com.

This primer is dedicated
to all those seeking assistance and support
on their journey to better breast health.
With deep gratitude we thank all those patients
who have obtained our services,
allowed us to learn through their experiences,
and encouraged us to develop this material.

Endorsements

I had recently been diagnosed with breast cancer, and felt my life was out of control. Better Breast Health - for Life! made me feel more in charge and in control of my situation. The details about food choices, personal products, and items we use in everyday life led me to make better decisions to support my health during and after my cancer treatment.

— **Glenna Biehler, age 37**

Excluding radiation and medications following my breast cancer surgery was a giant step for me, but for me, natural and alternative are my only options. I take comfort in the knowledge I have gained from Better Breast Health - for Life! and the increased sense of control I have in my healing process.

— **Helen Eisner, age 71**

I appreciated all the information in Better Breast Health - for Life! It is so encouraging to be able to make life changes with this knowledge. Finding out about all the risk factors from genetics to lifestyle is so helpful. The importance of exercise was particularly motivating to me. I now bounce on a fitness ball or trampoline. I love bouncing so this is a win-win for me!

— **Marilyn Fleming, age 68**

We all want to live in the communities of our choosing. While we can't always control every element of our environment or lives, this book gives me the information I need to make informed choices – to make changes within my comfort zone to lower my overall breast cancer risk. I really appreciate the workshop CD and worksheets. Now I have a prioritized list of the risk factors that are in my life and ways to exert some control!

— **Laura Sanchez, age 45**

It is timely indeed to have a consolidated information source for healthy breast awareness. This group of authors has dedicated their efforts to provide a desirable format of information, and to introduce thermal imaging as a way of monitoring and ensuring that preventative measures are effective! Thank you all for advancing healthy breast awareness for women!

— **Helen Taylor, age 52**

Contents

Acknowledgments

This publication will help many women because many caring individuals contributed to its development. First, there are the health professionals, whose years of experience and unique breast health specialties have been so crucial (in alphabetical order): Deborah Breakell, FNP, for ensuring that its medical terminology is accurate and straightforward; Carrie Louise Daenell, ND, whose dedication and generous contribution of time and effort have helped broaden its appeal; Carol Dalton, WHNP, for softening the sharp edges of its text; John RM Day, MD for his constant encouragement, support, and guidance; Tirza Derflinger, Founder, CTT, MBA-MOT for the passion and determination to ensure its completion; Lisa High, MS, RD, for a steady supply of the latest information on nutrition; and Kelly McAleese, MD, whose experiences with women's imaging and radiology have added tremendous benefit, accuracy, and validity.

Together, we constitute the Breast Health Education Group, authors of Better Breast Health – *for Life!*™ We owe thanks and recognition to our many supporters.

To all of the patients and their family members who have graciously shared their life experiences and requests for information with us; your input has shaped the contents and topics of this publication. Special thanks go out to Lynda Conis, Suzanne DeLucia, Helen Eisner, Marilyn Fleming, Jackie Logan, our proof-readers.

Additional thanks are extended to the health food stores/ companies that have sponsored and supported the years of breast health lectures that evolved into this publication: Vitamin Cottage (and Cindy Key), Whole Foods, and Wild Oats.

Finally, we thank our family and friends who have supported this endeavor, even though it often competed with family time.

We are grateful for each other, and each and every one of you.

Introduction

Do you know just how much control you have over your breast health? This question is the subject of Better Breast Health – *for Life!*™ The title itself conveys two messages. The first suggests that **better breast health supports life**. The second suggests that better breast health is a journey... one that lasts a lifetime.

It is our genuine intention that as you experience this material you feel energized and empowered to take charge of more of the risk factors for which you have some control. While it may not be practical or possible to manage all of the factors in your life, reducing just one influential factor may have positive and long-lasting effects. On the other hand, it is important to acknowledge that in spite of our best efforts, some breast cancers will occur. In these instances, regular breast screening and early detection are critical.

Part One explores how breast cancer develops and the methods and importance of early detection. Part Two explains the risk factors that contribute most to the disease by category: **genetic, estrogenic, environmental, health & lifestyle, and dietary**, and what you can do to reduce these risk factors in your life.

Part Three reveals a method to assess the collective effect of risk factors on your current breast health – **breast thermography**. Part Four includes the personal journeys of three women in breast health, and additional and on-line breast health resources and reference materials.

Also included with this material is a one-hour audio workshop CD, complete with worksheets. With these, you can **attend our Better Breast Health – *for Life!*™ Workshop – without leaving home!**

We encourage you to complete the workshop and "Risk Factors Worksheet" before reviewing the book. (This worksheet is shown on the following page.) Doing so will enable you **to identify and prioritize the risk factors present in *your* life**. Then you can focus on *your* highest priorities, learning how to impact them by referring to the contents of this book. Afterwards, you can use the "Actions Checklist" in the Summary Chapter (also on the CD) to record and track the action steps you have selected for yourself.

To listen to the audio CD, simply insert your CD into any CD player. To obtain full-size (8.5"x11") worksheets, insert the CD into your computer CD driver and use your file directory software and printer to open and print the "Risk Factors Worksheet" and "Actions Checklist" documents.

For your convenience, the websites listed in the following text are available as hotlinks on the CD. Use your file directory software to open the "Website" document on the CD. Each website is listed there in the order it appears in the following text. Just click on the website link of your choice to launch the website. (Requires an active Internet connection.)

This worksheet is intended to be used with the Better Breast Health - *for Life!*™ Audio Workshop CD and is designed to help you identify and prioritize areas of opportunity to reduce risk.

Areas of Opportunity & Risk Factors for Which Women Have Some Control (in the order each appears in the book, Better Breast Health - *for Life!*™)		Level of Added Risk
	Prolonged or Continuous:	
Genetics & Estrogen	waist to hip ratio greater than .81	H
	Body Mass Index over 25	L to M
	* no full-term pregnancy	L
	* using HRT or estrogen useage now and have been for at least 5 years	L
	* used birth control pills for at least 5 years prior to first full term pregnancy	M to H
	* premature delivery before 32 weeks	L
	* termination of teenage pregnancy between weeks 9 and 24	EH
	improper estrogen metabolism or estrogen dominance	L
Environment	toxin or carcinogen exposure, i.e agricultural and petro-chemicals	H
	pollutant or chemical exposure, i.e. non-natural personal or home cleaning products	L to M
	radiation exposure to breasts aged 8-20 years old	L to M
	high-powered EMF (electromagmetic frequency) exposure	EH
Health & Lifestyle	irregular sleep patterns	L to M
	smoking of tobacco	L to M
	alcohol consumption of at least 10 drinks/week	L to M
	drink only small amount of pure water daily (far less than 1/2 oz/lb of body weight)	N
	lack of sufficient sunlight	L
	deep, long-lasting emotional trauma/stress	N
	low to moderate daily stress levels	L
	high daily stress levels	M
	wearing bras more than 12 hrs/day, everyday, particularly if not professionally "fitted"	M
	sedentary lifestyle with little or no exercise	L to M
	never cleanse bodily systems	N
	symptoms of chronic inflammation	L
	medication or drug use	L to M
	low iodine/underactive thyroid	L to M
Diet	diet is not organic or hormone free	N
	acidic diet vs alkaline diet	N
	cooked/refined diet vs raw diet	L
	low fiber diet, i.e. less than 30g per day	L
	majority of fat intake is not in the form of organic monounsaturated fats	L
	Omega 6:Omega 3 ratio approaching 20+:1	L
	diabetic or high glycemic (sugar/starch) diet and postmenopausal	L
	little or no nutritional supplementation	N
	microwaving as primary method of cooking	N

| N** = no clinical risk   L = Low; = 2X   M = Medium; > 2X and = 5X |
| H = High: > 5X and = 10X   EH = Extremely High; > 10X |

* These items represent typical lifetime events rather than prolonged or continuous situations.
** These items represent potential areas of opportunity to support good health, but have no clinically-established association with the development of breast cancer. These areas may be investigated in the future for their association with the development of breast cancer and added risk.

PART ONE

BREAST CANCER AND EARLY DETECTION

1

How Does Breast Cancer Develop?

Breast cancers typically begin in the cells of the breast ducts or milk glands, which are referred to as lobules. The ducts are the pathways that deliver milk from the milk glands to the nipple for breast feeding. Depending on factors like the health of the internal environment of the breasts, hormones, and hereditary influences, cancer can behave in a variety of ways.

For instance, cancer can remain **in situ**, which is to say that it remains confined to the immediate area where it began, whether this is in the ducts or the lobules themselves. When in the ducts, it is referred to as ductal carcinoma in situ, or DCIS, and when in the lobules, lobular carcinoma in situ, or LCIS. In either case, the cancer has not invaded surrounding breast tissue or other organs in the body and is referred to as pre-invasive cancer.

When a cancer breaks through the ducts or lobules to invade surrounding tissue, it is called an **invasive or infiltrating** cancer. If it makes its way into the lymphatic system, which collects waste products and toxins from the tissues and extracellular fluid, then the cancer can spread to the lymph nodes.

At this stage, it is known as **regional metastasis**. Once breast cancer spreads to the lymph nodes under the arm or under the sternum (breastbone), there is an increased chance that the cancer can spread to other organs of the body, known as **distant metastasis**.

For more information on all known breast cancer types, their frequency of occurrence, treatment, and prognoses, visit the American Cancer Society website www.cancer.org/docroot/CRI/content CRI_2_4_1X_What_is_breast_cancer_5.asp.

2

How is Breast Cancer Detected?

Before the advent of mammography, breast cancer detection was dependent upon self-exam and clinical palpation, where the fingers are used to study the texture of the breasts and to search for masses. **Mammography** is an x-ray based technology that can detect masses years earlier, when the size of a mass is too small to be felt by palpation.

Recent advancements in mammography are enabling the detection of smaller cancers and more in-situ cancers. (In situ cancers are pre-invasive cancers, confined to their immediate area of origin.) Mammograms also detect microcalcifications, deposits of calcium, which are not cancers themselves, but are occasionally present with in-situ cancers of the duct. Following mammograms that are either suspicious or not clearly normal, or for young women with dense breast tissue that can make mammograms difficult to read, ultrasounds are often performed.

Using high-frequency sound waves, **ultrasounds** can help distinguish the fluid versus solid characteristics of tissue and masses. This is important because cancerous, malignant tumors are solid filled while benign, non-cancerous cysts are fluid filled. (Some breast cysts can contain cancer, but this occurs rarely.) Dr. Kelly McAleese, profiled in the chapter, "About the Authors," is Medical

5

Director and Radiologist at The Women's Imaging Center in Denver, one of many comprehensive breast and imaging centers across the country offering mammograms, ductograms, ultrasounds, biopsies, and bone density testing.

Moving up in expense and sophistication are MRIs and PET scans. An **MRI** involves injection of a rare earth mineral, magnetic fields, and radio waves to help evaluate the extent and locations of breast cancer. A **PET scan** uses an injection of glucose with a radioactive component to observe the location of an invasive breast cancer and to help in staging the extent of the disease once diagnosed.

It's important to note that only the **histology lab** can diagnose breast cancer, by studying actual tissue obtained from the breast by **biopsy** or surgical procedure. All breast exams then, are looking for signs that cancer may be present.

Did you know that mammography is the only exam approved by the U.S. Food and Drug Administration (FDA) to screen for breast cancer in women with no symptoms of the disease? This is why our healthcare providers typically initiate breast screening with a mammogram. The other exams are FDA approved as *supplements*, not *replacements*, for mammograms.

It is unfortunate that nearly 40% of U.S. women aren't getting routine screening by mammogram and might be missing out on the **early detection** that can save lives.[1] We hope that through education, more women understand the importance of mammograms and the complementary role of other methods of breast imaging.

For more information on breast cancer detection and testing, visit the American Cancer Society website www.cancer.org/docroot/CRI/content/CRI_2_4_3X_How_is_breast_cancer_diagnosed_5.asp?rnav=cri.

PART TWO

WHAT FACTORS CONTRIBUTE TO THE DEVELOPMENT OF BREAST CANCER?

To enable breast cancer prevention, we first need to understand the **most-likely causes, or risk factors**, that contribute to its development and how women can reduce them. It would be helpful if there was some test that could assess their impact on our breast health... but more on that later. First, we'll explore the risk factors known to impact breast health.

As a reminder, we suggest that you complete your Risk Factors Worksheet with the one-hour audio CD before proceeding. Doing so will focus your attention and efforts on only those risk factors pertinent to you, and also aid in prioritizing your efforts to reduce them.

3

Genetic Factors

Have you heard of hereditary risk or genetic predisposition? You might be surprised to learn that **hereditary risk is one of the most over-estimated risk factors by women**. Some studies indicate that only 2-5% of breast cancers are linked to inherited genes.[2, 3]

While the risk of developing breast cancer is higher in women with an inherited gene, like **BRCA-1** and **BRCA-2,** the significance of this statistic is that potentially 95-98% of breast cancers are linked to other, more controllable risk factors. For more information on gene testing and the risk associated with these inherited genes, visit the National Cancer Institute website http://cis.nci.nih.gov/fact/3_62.htm.

While we may have less control over hereditary factors, we can better understand them and how they contribute to our own risk for developing breast cancer. For instance, from birth to age 40, the risk of developing breast cancer among white women is 1 in 100. But "cumulative" risk is defined as the lifetime risk of women who live to age 85, and this is 1 in 8 for white women.

Statistically, breast cancer is more prevalent in women over age 50 than women under age 50, and **risk increases with age**. Risk is slightly less for African-American, Hispanic, Asian/Pacific, and American Indian women. Men can get breast cancer too, but account for only 1% of all cases.

For women with no risk factors, their absolute risk may be closer to 1 in 100, or 1%. For women with risk factors, absolute risk increases, or multiplies. For instance, statistics indicate that women whose mothers were diagnosed with breast cancer may be at nearly two times the risk of women whose mothers were not diagnosed.[4, 5]

The older the mother when diagnosed, the lower the risk for the daughter. If only a woman's aunt or grandmother was diagnosed, then risk may increase one and a half times. If a woman's mother and a sister have been diagnosed, then her risk can increase up to five times.[6]

While risk factors multiply our absolute risk, they are not additive. That is, we cannot simply add the multiplying effect of each risk factor to obtain a total. It's more complicated than that. Each additional risk factor does increase our absolute risk, but in a compounded way rather than an additive way.

Other characteristics of genetics and the body linked to risk include **skin color and body size**. While Caucasian women are slightly more at risk for breast cancer than African-American women, African-American and minority women are more likely to die of the disease, partly because of socioeconomic conditions.[7, 8] Some women over 5'6" and 154lbs are up to 3.6 times the risk of women under 5'3" and 132lbs.[9] **Body shape and fat distribution** impact this.

You've probably heard about the apple versus pear shaped figure, and that cancer risk is higher when we are apple shaped. Our shape can also be measured by our waist-to-hip ratio. This ratio is determined by dividing the waist measurement by the hip measurement. If this ratio is greater than .81, risk may increase up to seven times.[9]

Another way of learning if you are at risk by body shape and size is with the Body Mass Index, or BMI. To determine if your BMI correlates to a higher risk of adverse effects on health, determine your body height in inches and your weight in pounds and then visit the National Cancer Institute website http://cis.nci.nih.gov/fact/3_70.htm.

Or, divide your body weight in kilograms by your height in meters, squared:

$$\frac{\text{Body weight (kg)}}{\text{Body height (m}^2)} = \frac{\text{pounds} / 2.2}{(\text{inches}*0.0254)^2} = \text{BMI}$$

For example, consider a 175lb woman who is 5ft 7in tall:

$$\frac{\text{Body weight (kg)}}{\text{Body height (m}^2)} = \frac{175 / 2.2}{(67*0.0254)^2} = \frac{79.55}{(1.70)^2} = \frac{79.55}{2.89}$$

$$\text{BMI} = 28$$

Maintaining a BMI under 25 through adulthood supports breast health.[10]

Some studies indicate that postmenopausal women 50lbs or more overweight can be 1.5 times more likely to develop breast cancer, especially if the majority of excess weight was added in adulthood. The fat cells in postmenopausal women are very efficient at converting certain hormones from our adrenal glands into estrogens, which we will now explore as our next risk factor.

4

Estrogenic Factors

While there is much to be learned about cancer, we know that it involves **uncontrolled cellular growth**. Growth occurs when cell's divide, where one cell divides to become two cells. Normal breast cells can progress to a state of overgrowth, referred to as **hyperplasia**. If this division results in unusual cells, then it is referred to as **atypical hyperplasia**.

Cancer can result if mutations occur during the cellular division process. Under certain circumstances, estrogen can stimulate the breast tissue to increase cellular division. This is why **prolonged exposure to *excess* estrogen is probably *the* most significant risk factor** currently known for developing breast cancer. Excess estrogen also promotes cellular growth in the reproductive organs, i.e. the ovaries, so it is a risk factor there as well.

Women who start menstruating before age 9, or experience menopause after age 55, or have a first child after age 40, or have no or few children are statistically at higher risk. In general, the shorter the duration between our first menstruation and our first full-term pregnancy, the lower our risk of breast cancer.

This happens because **breast cells begin to mature with each menstrual cycle, but cannot complete the process without a full-term pregnancy. Immature breast cells have unstable DNA** and are more susceptible to mutation and the cancer process. In contrast, mature cells have more stable DNA and are more resistant.[6, 11, 12]

Do you remember how old you were when you experienced your first menses, or period? Most U.S. women start menstruating near ages 11-12. But in prior centuries, especially in non-industrialized nations, the average age was 16-17 years.[13]

Increased numbers of menstrual cycles increase our lifetime exposure to estrogen. During each menstrual cycle, our estrogen levels change, and increase in preparation for ovulation. An additional five years of estrogen production can increase breast cancer risk, especially if no full-term pregnancy ensues.

According to Dr. Susan Love, author of *Dr. Susan Love's Breast Book*, women who take estrogen for 5 to10 years generally increase their risk of breast cancer up to 1.5 times.[6] This would suggest that taking estrogen may add slightly to our level of risk. In a large clinical trial of the Women's Health Initiative (WHI), launched in 1991, the use of estrogen among postmenopausal women indicated no increase in the risk of breast cancer.[14]

In contrast, another WHI clinical trial indicated that postmenopausal women who took both estrogen and progestin, a synthetic hormone similar to progesterone, experienced an increased risk of developing breast cancer and heart disease. As a result, the trial was stopped early (in July 2002) for safety concerns.[15]

Since then the U.S. Food and Drug Administration (FDA) has recommended that women discuss whether the benefits of taking estrogen and progestin outweigh the risks with their healthcare providers. In addition, the FDA recommends that if used, hormones should be taken "at the lowest doses for the shortest duration to reach treatment goals." [15]

Some of us will go through the change of life and experience uncomfortable symptoms like hot flashes, sleeplessness, and emotional stress. While some of our healthcare providers will offer **hormone replacement therapy, or HRT,** others will attempt diet and lifestyle changes with herbal support.

If these prove ineffective, or if our symptoms become intolerable or debilitating, these providers may also turn to HRT. The good news is that the risk associated with HRT decreases rapidly after treatment is completed. Because natural bio-identical hormones reduce the risk of side effects, some healthcare providers offer them rather than synthetic or animal-derived hormones.

For more information on the risks and benefits associated with menopausal hormone use, visit the National Cancer Institute website www.cancer.gov/clinicaltrials/digest-postmenopausal-hormone-use and the U.S. Food & Drug Administration website www.fda.gov/cder/drug/infopage/estrogens_progestins/default.htm.

Younger women often ask about **birth control pills** and breast cancer risk. Evidence suggests that the pill can reduce estrogen absorption and slightly lower risk if used after the first full-term pregnancy.

If used before pregnancy or under the age of 20, or for more than 5 years before the age of 35, however, one 1993 study suggests risk can increase up to ten times.[16] (It is important to note that earlier forms of birth control pills typically contained higher amounts of estrogens than the pills of today.)

Risk may increase in some non-full-term pregnancy woman because exposure to estrogen is increased with the use of the pill while the breast cells are immature and least resistant to mutation.

A 1996 analysis of worldwide epidemiologic data (that which deals with disease) conducted by the Collaborative Group on Hormonal Factors in Breast Cancer found that women who were current or recent users of birth control pills had only a slightly elevated risk of developing breast cancer. Additionally, their analysis revealed that after ten years of not using the pill, these women's risk of developing breast cancer returned to the same level of women who had never used the pill. [17]

When the pill is used after the age of 45, evidence suggests that pill users are at no more risk than women who had never used the pill.[18, 19] To explore birth control methods, visit the U.S. Food & Drug Administration websites www.fda.gov/opacom/lowlit/brthcon.html and www.fda.gov/fdac/features/1997/babytabl.html.

There is good news for mothers, especially nursing mothers. Evidence suggests that **women who nurse** for at least six months after the age of 20 can reduce their risk by 25%, as nursing promotes breast cell maturation.[20, 21] Women who have 5 or more children may have a 50% less risk of breast cancer than women with no children.[22]

In addition, **pregnancies that do not go full term may increase our risk**. During the first two trimesters, high estrogen levels stimulate cellular division in the breast and increase the number of immature breast cells. Only during the third trimester do these cells start maturing. Some studies suggest that premature deliveries before 32 weeks can increase breast cancer risk two times. One study suggests that if a teenage pregnancy is terminated between weeks 9 and 24, the chance of developing breast cancer in her lifetime can increase to 30%.[16]

If either of these two events are a part of a woman's past medical history, she can direct her focus on other controllable estrogenic factors, i.e. estrogen metabolism and balance, and consult with a functional medicine doctor for professional assistance.

Isn't it remarkable how influential this one hormone is on our risk? By now you're probably wondering where estrogens come from. **Sources of estrogen** (and its mimickers) beyond hormone replacement therapy and birth control pills include: the environment, our ovaries, the body's fat cells, our adrenal glands, and our diet, particularly non-organic meats and dairy products which often contain growth hormones.

Estrogen can be reduced in the body by strenuous physical activity, certain dietary components, specific nutriceuticals and pharmaceuticals, and menopause. Estrogens are metabolized, or broken down, by the liver into either beneficial cancer-fighting metabolites, or cancer-promoting metabolites.

Some women's health care specialists provide tests that determine how well a woman is metabolizing, or breaking down her estrogens, i.e. metabolite ratio tests. Colorado 's naturopathic physician Dr. Carrie Louise Daenell and nurse practitioners Deborah Breakell and Carol Dalton, profiled in the chapter, "About the Authors", may be similar to healthcare providers in your local area that provide this testing, along with testing for adrenal and ovarian hormones, and assistance to correct hormonal and metabolic imbalances.

How can we reduce our risk from excess exposure to estrogen or their cancer-promoting metabolites? One way is to add phytoestrogens or phytochemicals. **Phytoestrogens** are compounds found in plants that may act like the estrogen produced naturally in our bodies. For example, wild yams are rich in phytoestrogens. These weak estrogen-like compounds can attach to the estrogen receptor sites in the breasts, and block stronger cancer-promoting estrogens and xenoestrogens (chemicals that mimic estrogen) from attaching.

Phytochemicals are plant chemicals that have protective, disease-fighting qualities. Some favorably affect estrogen metabolism in the liver.[23, 24]

According to Dr. Susan Lark, author of multiple self-help books on women's health, phytochemicals like diindolylmethane (DIM), which is derived from the indole-3-carbinol found in vegetables like broccoli, bok choy, cauliflower, cabbage and brussels sprouts, can support normal estrogen metabolism for healthy breast tissue, potentially reducing the breast tenderness and mood swings associated with our menstrual cycles. [25]

In addition, she points out that glucarate, another phytochemical found in apples, apricots, cherries, broccoli, alfalfa sprouts, bean sprouts, and brussels sprouts supports the elimination of metabolized estrogens from the body through our bowels.

She adds that in the absence of glucuronic acid, which the body forms from glucarates, the liver cannot properly metabolize estrogens, and the body cannot eliminate estrogen through the bowels. Instead, estrogens can get reabsorbed from the intestines into the bloodstream, adding to the level of estrogen in the body.[25] (Increased fiber in the diet can also help reduce estrogen metabolite reabsorption from the bowels.)

While it can be helpful to support the liver's ability to metabolize estrogen and the body's ability to eliminate it, there are many herbs, phytonutrients, and nutritional supplements to consider. Consult with healthcare providers or functional medicine doctors who emphasize healthy estrogen metabolism in their practice when considering the need for metabolism support and the supplements that are right for you.

5

Environmental Factors

Now let's move on to the environment and how we ingest estrogens from it. Prior to World War II, there were limited **chemicals and pollution** in our environment and society. Today, the typical American is exposed to hundreds of chemicals each day. These chemicals can enter the body by way of ingestion, breathing, or skin penetration. Some of these chemicals can imitate estrogens, referred to as **xenoestrogens**, or disrupt our hormones and contribute to the risk of developing breast cancer.

Devra Lee Davis, Ph.D., a university researcher who served as a senior advisor to the Department of Health and Human Services, pointed to pesticides, household chemicals, and common plastics as the sources of xenoestrogens, few of which existed before World War II. She proposed that breast cancer may be caused by dozens of common, synthetic chemicals that mimic the female hormone estrogen: "If xenoestrogens do play a role in breast cancer, reductions in exposure will provide an opportunity for primary prevention of this growing disease."[26]

Handling and breathing **petroleum-based chemicals** like gasoline, kerosene, benzene, and formaldehyde, especially when burned, are known to induce cancers in the mammary glands of animals. Among postmenopausal women, breast cancer rates are statistically 1.6 times higher when living within one-half mile from a chemical plant.[27]

Agricultural chemicals like pesticides, herbicides, and fertilizers; also chlorinated water; many disinfectants; and plastics contain **organochlorines**. These are chlorine-based chemicals thought to contribute significantly to breast cancer. They can mutate genes, alter breast cells to absorb more estrogen, suppress the immune system, and can imitate the bad effects of estrogen.[28]

They can enter the body by way of drinking, showering, or swimming in chlorinated water; by eating food, meat, dairy, fruits, or vegetables produced with chemicals; by exposing the skin to chlorine-bleached products or personal hygiene products; or from certain plastics migrating into foods, especially those that involve heating or microwaving.

Organochlorines are metabolized in the liver and by processes supported by phytochemicals like diindolylmethane and glucarate derivatives. The size of organochlorine molecules however, makes metabolism more difficult, so the majority of them end up being stored in fat cells and in the breast tissue.

Some research indicates that women with breast cancer have 50-60% more organochlorine molecules in their tissues than women without breast cancer.[29, 30] After the nation of Israel banned several organochlorine pesticides, women's breast cancer mortality dropped by a third for women under the age of 44, demonstrating the link between environmental chemicals and increased rates of breast cancer mortality.[31]

To demonstrate the sometimes subtle effects of eating everyday, non-organic foods, consider another study in the medical journal *Lancet* which found that men who ate mostly pesticide-free organic foods had sperm concentrations 43% higher than men who ate a standard diet. [32]

We can reduce our exposure to organochlorines by 80% by eating organically produced animal products like eggs, milk, cheese, and meat, and by consuming organic produce and filtered water. Using less plastic and buying fresh versus canned or packaged pantry foods can help too. Since our skin is the body's largest organ, using all natural personal products, all natural household cleaners, and non-bleached paper products can also help.

When you think of **personal products**, be sure to think broadly and include items like skin and eye cosmetics, moisturizers, shaving creams, soaps, bubble bath, bath oils, shampoos, conditioners, mouthwash, toothpaste, sunscreen, antiperspirants and deodorants, perfumes and colognes, nail polish and remover, and other hair care products, including coloring. (Many natural health food stores offer "natural" personal products.)

Darker hair dye colors carry more risk than lighter colors, which is better news for those who want to be blondes. While deodorants act to deodorize perspiration, antiperspirants act to reduce it, which can reduce our ability to purge toxins.

Many non-natural personal products contain chemicals that are suspected carcinogens and/or toxins, contaminates, skin irritants, or **endocrine disruptors**. An endocrine disruptor is a synthetic chemical that when absorbed into the body either mimics or blocks hormones and disrupts normal body functions. For more information on endocrine disruptors visit the National Resources Defense Council website www.nrdc.org/health/effects/qendoc.asp#disruptor.

For a list of the top 40 potentially harmful ingredients commonly used in personal products, or to check the ingredients on the labels of your products, visit the website www.antiagingchoices.com/harmful_ingredients/toxic_ingredients.htm.

Dioxins are created in forest fires, cement kilns, coal burning power plants, the chlorine bleaching of wood pulp, and the burning of trash or firewood. They are transported primarily through the air and are commonly detected in air, soil, water, food, and in animal and human tissues in trace amounts. The Environmental Protection Agency indicates that they are highly toxic and a substance that is expected to increase the risk of cancer. Present in the water supply of most industrialized nations, dioxins are expected to double breast cancer risk.

We can reduce our exposure to dioxins in a variety of ways. Using filtered water rather than tap water can reduce the risk. Certain high-quality water and air filters can purify at a molecular level and are available in a variety of forms and through a variety of sources. For instance, water filters are available for sink faucets, refrigerator water lines, shower heads, and the main water supply for an entire dwelling. Similarly, high-quality whole-house and single-room air filters are also available.

Since organochlorine and endocrine disrupting chemicals can be released from plastics, especially when those plastics are exposed to microwaving, heat, or sunlight, heating and storing foods and water in glass, ceramics, or stainless steel can help reduce this risk.

Another way to reduce chemical exposure is to use the right plastic for the right purpose when glass, ceramics, and stainless steel are not an option. Heat, fat, and extended use all speed up the chemical leaching process in plastics. We should not microwave plastic that's not specified for such use (such as margarine tubs) or put top-shelf-only plastics, such as children's sippy cups and baby bottles, on the bottom shelf of a dishwasher. If a plastic container starts to look cloudy or scratchy, or has an odor to it, dispose of it or recycle it.[32]

Most water, soda, juice, and sports-drink bottles, yogurt cartons, bread bags, boil-in-bag pouches, cereal-box liners, and food-storage bags are examples of food-grade plastics with no known health hazards when they are not exposed to heat.[32] (However, these containers are generally intended for single use, i.e. #1 PET or PETE, and should be discarded after their initial use rather than cleaned and re-used.)

In general, the more flexible the plastic, the more likely it is to contain plasticizers like phthalates, which make plastic more pliable. While some phthalates are harmless, others may contribute to cancer.

Endocrine disrupting chemicals, **phthalates** can migrate from plastics, especially in the presence of heat. Being fat soluble, phthalates can concentrate in the fatty organs of our bodies, including the breasts. A recent study published in *Environmental Health Perspective* also links the irregular genital development in boys of mothers exposed to multiple phthalates during pregnancy. [33]

Many polyvinyl chloride products, #3 PVC, and food containers, plastic wrap, styrofoam cups, soft vinyl products and toys, baby bottles, and plastic teethers, contain phthalates.[32]

Another endocrine disruptor is **bisphenol-A**. According to *Endocrinology*, "Humans are exposed to bisphenol-A (BPA), an estrogenic compound that leaches from dental materials and plastic food and beverage containers." [34] Animal experiments have linked bisphenol-A to an increased risk for breast and prostate cancer, low sperm counts, and female infertility at very low levels of exposure. [35] Some polycarbonate plastics, #7 PC, found in food can linings, baby bottles, 5-gallon water jugs, and Lexan or Nalgene water bottles contain bisphenol-A.[32]

To be safe, experts suggest beverage and baby bottles made of stainless-steel, glass, or plastics not known to leach harmful substances: [36]

- Polypropylene, #5 PP
- High-density polyethylene, #2 HDPE
- Low-density polyethylene, #4 LDPE

For purchase information on beverage bottles made exclusively of these plastic materials, visit the Blender Bottle website www.blenderbottle.com.

For purchase information on polypropylene baby bottles made by Medela and their Day Carrier Kit, visit the Amazon website www.shopping.com/xFS?KW=Medela+ Accessories&FN=Baby+Care&FD=85708 or the Baby Mania website www.breastfeedingaccessories.com/cooler_ carriers.html.

While glass, ceramic, and stainless steel make relatively safe storage and cooking containers, waxed-paper sheets and bags, and parchment paper can substitute for plastic wraps and bags.[32]

For a list of known environmental pollutants and toxins from the Environmental Protection Agency, visit www.epa.gov/ebtpages/pollutants.html.

For a Citizen's Guide to Pest Control and Pesticide Safety, visit www.epa.gov/oppfead1/Publications/Cit_Guide/citguide.pdf.

For the latest Report on Carcinogens from the Department of Health and Human Services, visit www.nih.gov/news/pr/jan2005/niehs-31.htm.

For the Environmental Working Group's study on the toxic effect of various chemicals in our food supply, visit www.foodnews.org/effects.php.

For a list of environmental pollutants and toxins from the National Institutes of Health, visit http://ntp.niehs.nih.gov/index.cfm?objectid=72016262-BDB7-CEBA-FA60E922B18C2540.

Our next environmental factor is **radiation** exposure. There are many facts and myths around this topic, so let's try to make sense of them. When we measure radiation exposure, we use the unit of measure called a millirad (mrad). For example, one week of living at high altitude in Denver presents about 1 mrad of radiation while a 6 hour jet flight presents about 5 mrads, and a screening mammogram presents about 300 mrad. [28]

While the dense breast tissue among younger, premenopausal women requires about twice the radiation of their postmenopausal counterparts with less dense tissue, this should not cause concern. For perspective, external beam radiation treatment for breast cancer typically involves over 2,000,000 mrad.[37] Further, there are only a few circumstances in which mammography is known to increase risk.

Risk is substantially increased if radiation is absorbed in the developing breast tissue of women aged 8-20 years.[38] In these women, and in those women who are sensitive to radiation, (these women become physically ill after exposure) low level accumulation can increase risk and initiate cancer, appearing 10 years after exposure and not peaking until 40 years after exposure.[39, 40] However, for non-sensitive women over the age of 40, the added risk of mammography is statistically insignificant.

Another environmental risk comes with electric and **electromagnetic fields, or EMF**. These are the invisible lines of force that surround any electrical device. While they are a part of our everyday lives, constant exposure increases breast cancer rates.

For example, evidence suggests that women who work with telephone line installation or repair are up to 200 times more likely to develop breast cancer.[41] EMF can disturb the normal growth of cells by interfering with their hormone, enzyme, and chemical signals, causing DNA damage, and the potential for cancer.

EMF also reduces production of **melatonin**, a brain chemical that contributes to breast cancer when it is in a state of deficiency. (This is also why some flight attendants have higher incidence rates of breast cancer, not because of radiation exposure, but because their irregular sleep patterns disturb their melatonin levels.[42])

Computer monitors typically emit electric and magnetic fields in the very low frequency (VLF), and extremely low frequency (ELF) ranges. For women who sit in front of computer monitors during their work days, grounded glare screen filters are available to reduce the electric fields. Reducing the magnetic fields requires additional equipment to surround and shield the top and sides of the monitor. Flat screen monitors such as liquid crystal displays, or LCDs, and plasma displays, typically emit less EMF than do cathode ray tube, or CRT, monitors.

You'll be glad to know that **we can reduce the power of EMF from common household appliances by 80%** by keeping our bodies at least 28" away from electric clocks, electric wiring, TVs, computer monitors, electric blankets, electric fans, and other common household electric appliances. Hair dryers and bedside clocks can do more damage than TVs because they are typically closer to the head and the glands that regulate melatonin and other hormones. For more info on EMF, visit the National Cancer Institute website http://cis.nci.nih.gov/fact/3_46.htm.

6

Health & Lifestyle Factors

Now that we have explored environmental factors, let's look at another category of risk factors that we have even more control over. These are the risk factors associated with our health and lifestyles.

It's no surprise that **smoking and drinking** impact our breast health. But you may be surprised to learn why. Commercial **cigarettes**, grown with chemical fertilizers, can contain not only organochlorines, but also two radioactive elements, lead and polonium, which can contribute significantly to breast and lung cancers. Combustion of chlorine-bleached cigarette paper is also cancer-causing.

Studies suggest that risk increases with the number of years and the number of cigarettes smoked, with risk increases varying from .04 times to 4 times. Active smokers typically heal more slowly following surgery, experience more side effects from chemotherapy, and are more likely to die from breast cancer than non-smoking women.[43] Sufficient second hand smoke is also known to cause cancer, but is not linked to an increased risk for breast cancer.

Alcohol in the blood results in less melatonin production and more cancer-promoting estrogen metabolites out of the liver, especially in premenopausal and pre-first full-term pregnancy women.[44, 45] Studies vary on the increase in risk associated with varying levels of drinking, from increased risk at four alcoholic drinks a week to a 2.5 times increase at two drinks daily.

For breast health, consider eliminating or limiting alcohol consumption, drinking in moderation, and/or drinking organic wines and beers. If you do choose to drink, consider consulting with a specialist to design a liver supporting nutritional regimen specific to your needs.

Speaking of drinking, you may be aware of the importance of **water and hydration**. Did you know that the body is made up of at least 70% water? Involved in every bodily function, water enables the body to transport nutrients and flush out toxins and waste products. Drinking one half to one ounce of pure water for each pound of body weight each day helps the body stay adequately hydrated.

This means that a 120lb woman, for example, should drink 60-120 ounces of pure water each day. Pure or filtered water, versus tap water, is best. Pure water can be sourced from artesian wells or springs without added ingredients, outside of antimicrobial agents.

Colorado's Eldorado Springs is one of the purest waters in the world. Reverse osmosis is very effective for filtering heavy metals, uranium, chlorine, and fluoride. Steam distilled water is pure too, but some experts believe that it should not be consumed for prolonged periods since it leaches minerals from the body, and this can contribute to reduced bone density, and its medical term, osteoporosis, among many other mineral-deficient disease states. Fresh organic fruits and vegetables with natural juices are other sources of healthful liquids, as are broth soups, salsas, and other fluid-rich foods.

Sufficient sunlight is important for the body's production of **vitamin D**, which helps to strengthen the immune system and may help to prevent some types of cancer. Vitamin D is formed naturally when skin is exposed to sunlight. Women who live in sunnier parts of the U.S. or in the southern hemisphere have statistically reduced risk of breast cancer.[46]

In latitudes around 40 degrees north or south of the equator (Sacramento is 38° north while Denver is 39° north, and New York City is 40° north), there is insufficient ultraviolet-B radiation for vitamin D synthesis from November to early March. At locations further north or south of this latitude the "vitamin D winter" is extended.

According to Dr. Michael Holick at the Mayo Clinic, 5-10 minutes of sun exposure on arms and legs or face and arms (bare and without sunscreen) three times a week between the hours of 11 am and 2 pm during the spring, summer, and fall within 42 degrees latitude of the equator should provide a light-skinned individual with adequate vitamin D. (Dark-skinned individuals typically require additional sunlight exposure.) [47]

Because sunlight won't be sufficient at certain times of the year or in certain places, and because the body's ability to manufacture vitamin D declines with age, some people may need to get more vitamin D through foods, like fortified milk, fatty fish, and fish oils, or nutritional supplements. Since vitamin D can become toxic if consumed in excess, consult with a nutritional specialist to determine if you are deficient, and the form of supplementation and total daily amount that is appropriate for you. For more information on sunlight and vitamin D, visit the Oregon State University Linus Pauling Institute Micronutrient Information Center at http://lpi. oregonstate.edu/infocenter/vitamins/vitaminD/.

What about **stress**? It contributes to many disorders by increasing production of certain hormones, by creating nutritional deficiencies, and by compromising the immune system. A study published in 1995 in the *British Medical Journal* indicates that for women who experience stress-inducing events like job loss, bereavement, or divorce, risk may increase 12 times for the five year period following the event. [48]

According to the National Cancer Institute, some studies suggest higher rates of breast cancer among women who experience traumatic life events and losses. Although these studies have shown that such stress factors alter the way the immune system functions, more research is needed to substantiate a direct cause-and-effect relationship between immune system changes and the development of breast cancer.

For twenty years, Dr. John R.M. Day was a breast surgeon in Boulder, Colorado. One common thread among all the women he encountered with breast cancer was that each had experienced some **emotional heart-felt trauma**, usually in a 2 to 5 year period prior to the cancer diagnosis. He suspects that unresolved traumas related to experiences of grief can negatively impact the energy field around the heart and contribute to the development of breast cancer.

Today he works as a certified holistic practitioner and helps women to resolve old emotional and physical traumas, and to develop healthy nutrition and exercise regimens, mental and emotional clarity, self love, spiritual awareness and alignment, and vision for life goals. He is profiled in the chapter, "About the Authors" in the event you choose to seek a similar specialist in your local area.

Dr. Christiane Northrup, author of *Women's Bodies, Women's Wisdom* and *The Wisdom of Menopause,* indicates that there is a connection between our emotional and physical beings by way of chakras. **Chakras** are the seven energy centers in the body that, according to her, "connect our nerves, hormones, and emotions… and run parallel to the body's neuroendocrine-immune system…"[48]

Each chakra, or energy center, has been linked to specific organs of the body by Eastern cultures. The fourth chakra, located between the breasts, is the chakra linked to the breasts. In the book *Women's Bodies, Women's Wisdom,* Carolyn Myss, a renowned medical intuitive notes that the major emotions behind breast cancer are "hurt, sorrow, and unfinished emotional business generally related to nurturance." [48]

The energy center that can store the emotions of a "broken heart", the fourth chakra, according to Dr. Northrup, can contribute to ill health when we have issues with fully expressing and resolving anger, hostility, joy, love, grief, and forgiveness. [48]

It seems logical then, that developing positive, supportive emotional and spiritual relationships and maintaining appropriate, effective methods of self-expression can be helpful. Surrounding oneself with love from others, self-love, and laughter may also add to well being.

It's no surprise that stress comes in many forms, including physical, psychological, emotional, social, mental, and financial. Worry, overwork, change, deadlines, crowds, traffic, and excess noise create stress. Let's face it, stress is a part of our everyday lives, so learning to relax and reduce stress supports good health.

Sufficient sleep, exercise, meditation, yoga, deep breathing, living with pets, and quieting the noise in our minds are just a few of the many ways that people address their stress levels. What's important is to identify the healthy stress-reducers that work for you.

Women often ask about **bras**. Many younger women are wearing panties and bras 24/7 as part of a fashion trend. One study suggests that women who wear bras for more than 12 hours a day increase their risk by 6 times, while going generally braless reduces risk by 20 times.[49]

This applies to small and large women alike, though some very large breasted women have a need to wear their bra constantly for support. The good news for them is that the effect of their bra is spread out over a large surface area. In particular, the elastic in bras can hinder immune response and slow lymphatic circulation. While underwire bras can magnify these problems, properly fitted bras help reduce the risk.

Each year, Nordstrom stores sponsor Fit For The Cure, in which $2 is donated to the Susan Komen Foundation for each woman who is fitted during this event. For more information on a Fit for The Cure event near you, contact a store near you or visit www.nordstrom.com. Of course, women can be properly fitted outside of this event by trained staff members at Nordstrom or other upscale department stores.

You may be asking about the term, lymphatic circulation. If you recall from Chapter 1 about how breast cancer develops, the lymphatic system, with its highway of vessels and nodes, extracts waste products and toxins from the tissues and extracellular fluids. Therefore, it is important that lymphatic pathways remain unobstructed.

Exercise helps to move and clear the **lymphatic system**. The by-product of exercise, sweating, enables toxins and waste products to leave the body through the sweat glands. Unlike the circulation system which has its own pump called the heart, the lymphatic system has no pump. The body must move to stimulate the circulation of lymph fluid.

One of the best **exercises to stimulate lymph fluid circulation** involves an up and down motion, like that obtained while riding a horse, jumping on a mini-trampoline, or bouncing while sitting on a fitness ball.

Deep breathing, lymph massage, manual lymph pumping techniques, certain herbs and formulas, and dry brushing followed by a hot shower in which the last two minutes is in cold water are other common ways of stimulating lymphatic system circulation. For more information on lymphatic health, clearing congestion, or the clearing techniques which are right for you, consult with a lymphatic therapist or an informed healthcare provider.

As you probably know, **exercise** supports good health in many ways. Aerobic, range-of-motion, and/or strengthening exercise can: improve digestion and elimination; increase endurance and energy levels; deliver oxygen to the blood and tissues; promote lean body mass while burning fat; improve cholesterol levels; reduce blood pressure, stress and anxiety; increase perspiration; promote restful sleep; and elevate mood and the sense of well-being!

What's important to know is that regular and moderate exercise can be very healthful for women, decreasing estrogen production and enhancing estrogen metabolism.

The American Cancer Society reports that one study found that as little as 1 ¼ to 2 ½ hours per week of brisk walking reduced risk by 18%. Walking 10 hours a week reduced the risk a little more. Some other studies indicate that by exercising at least 4 hours a week, young women can reduce their risk of breast cancer 37-60%. The highest reductions are found among pre-menopausal women rather than post-menopausal women.[6, 50, 51]

Exercise can include yoga, dance, weight lifting, walking, just to name a few. Please note: over-exercise can become a stress on the body with negative impacts like amenorrhea, the absence of menstrual bleeding.

In addition to clearing lymphatic pathways, **cleansing body systems** is also an important aspect of good health. While there are many cleansing techniques, we'll explain some body-basics to help you understand the choices.

The lymphatic system filters wastes and toxins from the tissues and extracellular fluids. Resulting filtrates are carried through the bloodstream to the spleen and the liver, which processes them into fat soluble and water soluble components. These are components that dissolve in fat, and components that dissolve in water, respectively. The water soluble components re-enter the bloodstream and are filtered by the kidneys for elimination from the body through the urine. The fat soluble components are passed from the liver to the colon through bile secretion. (For more info on the lymphatic system visit Wikipedia's on-line encyclopedia at http://en.wikipedia.org/wiki/Lymphatic_system.)

When the colon has sufficient fiber, adequate levels of friendly bacteria, like Lactobacilli, and is not congested or dehydrated, then elimination of wastes and toxins is facilitated. But if insufficient fiber, inadequate bacteria levels, or dehydration exists in the colon, the components can be reabsorbed into the blood stream. It is possible that the entire process can back up and lead to inflammation, toxicity, and auto-immune disorders. Do you have as many bowel movements in a day as you have meals in a day? If not, there may be an opportunity for cleansing and improved bowel health.

While **clearing, cleansing, and supporting the colon** are helpful for enabling clearing and cleansing of the liver, lymphatic system, and bloodstream, again, please consult with an informed healthcare provider when considering colon health or the cleansing regimen that's right for you.

In addition to stress, factors like prolonged alcohol, drug and marijuana use, chemotherapy, toxic metals, negative emotions, an underactive thyroid, and inadequate nutrition can also effect the liver 's ability to metabolize estrogens, reduce the body's ability to eliminate undesirable components, and compromise the immune system.

Signs of a **compromised immune system** include chronic or frequent infections or colds, asthma, rheumatoid arthritis, allergies, chronic fatigue and fibromyalgia. These signs can also suggest chronic levels of inflammation.

Chronic inflammation arises when the immune system is constantly "on". That is, inflammation is a normal response to health issues like infections, but when the immune system doesn't turn off, it can remain hyper-active and contribute to chronic levels of inflammation and increased risk for breast cancer.

Common signs of potential inflammation in the digestive tract include bloating, gas or pain, frequent diarrhea or constipation, and heartburn or acid reflux. Because improper digestion can be linked to hormonal imbalances, immune disorders, and chronic inflammation, holistic healthcare providers like Deb Breakell and Carol Dalton, and naturopathic physicians like Dr. Carrie Louise Daenell (each featured in the chapter, "About the Authors") use natural and nutritionally-based methods to safeguard against the inflammation process, and to resolve its underlying causes.

What about using **prescription medications**? Did you know that they can increase our cancer risk when used for extended periods of time? For instance, beta-blockers that treat high blood pressure also suppress melatonin production, which contributes to breast cancer when in a state of deficiency.

Virtually all prescription medications work paradoxically, aiding in some ways while depleting nutrients in the body and increasing our cancer risk. The list includes anti-depressants, steroids, cortisones, diuretics, antihistamines, and statins, just to name a few. For more information, consult the *Drug-Induced Nutrient Depletion Handbook* available through book retailers and libraries. [52] For example:

Prescription Category	**Nutrient Depletions**
Estrogens (Hormone Replacement Therapy)	calcium, coenzyme $Q_{10,}$ folic acid, magnesium, vitamin B_6
Oral Contraceptives	folic acid, magnesium, Selenium, vitamins $B_{1,}$ $B_{2,}$ $B_{3,}$ $B_{6,}$ $B_{12,}$ vitamin C, and zinc

If you are using prescription medications, consult with your healthcare provider about their contributions to increased risk and the possibility of adding nutritionally-supportive therapies.

Also, consider consulting with a qualified natural healthcare provider on natural alternatives and supportive therapies. These providers may seek to remedy the underlying cause of the symptoms and resolve the need for medications altogether.

Did you know that there is a link between **our teeth and our breasts**? According to Chinese medicine, there are meridians, invisible channels through which chi, a form of life-force energy, circulates throughout the body. Root canals performed in teeth whose meridians are linked to the breasts, primarily the 3rd and 4th molars from the back of each jaw, have been linked to increased risk of breast cancer.[53] To reduce this risk, some women seek to extract the tooth *and* its periodontal ligament instead of undergoing a root canal.

Heavy metals and silver amalgam dental fillings have also been linked to a weakened immune system. Amalgam fillings are comprised of approximately 50% mercury, which can slowly bleed out of the fillings, concentrating in the liver, kidneys, brain, and other glands. Roughly 25% of the mercury in amalgam fillings can bleed out in the first five years, and the mercury vapor level in a mouth with amalgams can be 54 times higher than that in a mouth without amalgams.[54] According to a study at the University of Tennessee, mercury is second only to radioactive plutonium on the toxic scale of heavy metals.

There are many other **sources of mercury** besides amalgam fillings. Did you know that fish are often high in mercury? They're actually a controlled substance in grade schools, which are required to limit the number of servings of tuna due to its high mercury levels.[55]

According to the U.S. Food and Drug Administration and the Environmental Protection Agency, the risk from mercury by eating fish and shellfish is not a health concern for most people. However they advise women who may be pregnant, pregnant women, and young children to avoid some types of fish and to eat fish and shellfish that are lower in mercury: [56]

- Do not eat shark, swordfish, king mackerel, or tilefish, which contain high levels of mercury.
- Eat no more than 12 ounces per week of fish and shellfish that are lower in mercury: shrimp, canned light tuna (not albacore tuna), salmon, pollock, and catfish.
- Consult local authorities or www.epa.gov/water science/fish/states.htm for advisories on contaminated or polluted fishing areas and about the safety of fish from local lakes, rivers, and coastal areas.

For more information on mercury, consider visiting the Environmental Protection Agency, the Environmental Working Group, and the Audubon Society websites www.epa.gov, www.ewg.org, and www.audubon.org. For more information on bio-friendly dental procedures and the removal of amalgam fillings, consult with biological or environmental dentists.

The herb cilantro helps the body to eliminate mercury. Many oral and intravenous chelating processes can help too. **Chelating** refers to a substance that binds with, say a heavy metal, to neutralize its bad effect on the body and to facilitate the body's ability to eliminate it.

Since not everyone with amalgam fillings has unstable mercury in their fillings or mercury that needs to be chelated, and since ingesting too much cilantro can cause digestive symptoms, please consult with a qualified healthcare provider when considering the need for chelation and the technique that is right for you.

Some specialized healthcare providers, like Dr. Carrie Louise Daenell, provide a non-invasive genetic test to determine if a person is genetically predisposed and less able to eliminate mercury from the body, as is the case for a certain percentage of the population. For these individuals, customized nutritional protocols can be established to support this compromised process.

Our last health factor involves **iodine and thyroid hormones**. When in proper balance, each of these generally reduce the risk of breast cancer. On the other hand, iodine deficiency during puberty can produce the overgrowth of cells in breast tissue that can contribute to cancer risk.

Breast cancer rates are generally higher in regions of the world where iodine is deficient in the soil. Low iodine levels in the body reduce thyroid function, whereas high levels of iodine can help treat breast cancer.[57] Seaweed is an excellent source of iodine and is believed to contribute to Japan's low rate of breast cancer.

It also supports recovery for radiation patients, as does chlorophyll from algae, alfalfa, wheat and barley grasses, and other leafy green vegetables. Be aware that excess iodine can wreak havoc on the thyroid as well, so it is important to consult with a qualified healthcare provider when considering an increase in iodine consumption or its supplementation and to learn about tests to see if you are iodine deficient.

7

Dietary Factors

Besides **organic food and drink**, there are many other dietary factors that contribute to breast health. One example is **an alkaline diet**, which has to do with how our bodies digest foods and the impact of digestion on our blood pH, or the resulting level of acidity or alkalinity in the blood.

Hippocrates was a great Greek physician who some recognize as the father of medicine. He practiced the **80/20 principle**, professing that a diet comprised of 80% alkalizing foods and 20% acidifying foods supports good health. He also increased the proportion of alkalizing foods in times of health crises. The premise is that most viruses, bacteria, molds, fungus and yeast require an acidic environment and cannot survive in blood - or breast tissue - that is alkaline.

Foods that tend to support an alkaline pH include fruits that are acidic to the mouth, like: lemons, limes, grapefruit, and tomatoes, as well as almonds, avocados, cucumbers, strawberries, watermelon, most fruits and vegetables, and buckwheat and millet flours. Acidifying foods include all meats, which require a substantial amount of hydrochloric acid in the stomach to be digested, along with most dairy products, alcohol, commercial coffees, soft drinks, flours, and sugars.

We have provided a quick-reference alkaline/acidic food chart below:

Common Acid Categories		Common Alkaline Categories	
Alcohol	Nuts, Most	Flours (buckwheat and millet)	
Coffees	Poultry	Fruits, Most	
Dairy, Most	Soda/Soft Drinks	Nuts, Some	
Fish, All	Sugars	Sprouted Nuts & Seeds	
Flours, Most	Overcooked Foods, All	Vegetables, Most	
Meats, All	Unsprouted Nuts & Seeds		

Common Acid Foods

Bacon	Olives
Beans	Organ Meats
Beef	Oysters
Bran, Wheat	Peanut Butter
Bran, Oats	Peanuts
Bread, White	Peas, Dried
Bread, Wheat	Poultry
Carob	Plums
Catsup	Pork
Cheese	Prunes
Chicken	Refined Sugar
Cocoa	Salmon
Coffee	Sardines
Cod Fish	Sausage
Corn Starch	Scallops
Corn Oil	Shrimp
Corn Syrup	Soft drinks
Coconut	Sugar
Corned Beef	Squash, Winter
Crackers, Soda	Sunflower Seeds
Cranberries	Tea
Currants	Turkey
Eggs	Veal
Fish	Vegetable Oil
Flour, White	Walnuts
Flour, Wheat	Water, Tap
Haddock	Wheat Germ
Ice Cream	Yogurt
Lamb	
Legumes	**Better Acid Foods**
Lobster	Barley
Milk, Cow	Blueberries
Meat	Corn
Mustard	Honey
Nuts, Most	Lentils, Dried

Oatmeal
Olive Oil
Pasta
Rice, all

Neutral Foods

Butter
Water, Distilled

Alkaline Foods

Almonds	Grapes
Amaranth	Green Beans
Apples	Green Peas
Apricots	Lemons
Avocados	Lettuce
Bananas	Lima Beans, Dried
Beet Greens	Lima Beans, Green
Beets	Limes
Buckwheat	Milk, Goat
Buckwheat Flour	Millet
Blackberries	Millet Flour
Broccoli	Molasses
Brussel Sprouts	Mushrooms
Brazil Nuts	Onions
Cabbage	Oranges
Cantalope	Parsnips
Carrots, Sweet-	Peaches
Cauliflower	Pears
Celery	Pineapple
Chard Leaves	Potatoes, Sweet
Cherries, Sour	Potatoes, White
Chestnuts	Quinoa
Cucumbers	Radishes
Dates, Dried	Raspberries
Figs, Dried	Rutabagas
Grapefruit	Sauerkraut
	Soy Beans, Green
	Sea Vegetables
	Spinach, Raw
	Sprouts
	Strawberries
	Tangerines
	Tomatoes
	Watercress
	Watermelon

You can also visit the alkaline/acidic food charts at www.essense-of-life.com/info/foodchart.htm. However, some people do not metabolize foods according to these generalized charts. To learn which foods typically result in alkalinity or acidity in your body, please consult with a provider of metabolic typing, as each of the nine different metabolic types affects the way each body metabolizes food. You can also visit the on-line metabolic typing questionnaire at www.metabolictyping.com.

By now you may have surmised that the typical American diet is acidifying… especially fast foods, often made up of breads, meats, dairy, soft drinks, and processed packaged foods. In order for the blood to neutralize the acidifying effects of these foods, it acquires alkalizing minerals and calcium from the body.

Afterwards, these minerals do not return to the tissues or bone… they have been consumed. This process can contribute to osteoporosis, which takes more lives than uterine, ovarian, and breast cancers…combined. Now you understand why an alkaline diet is so very important as a basic fundamental to good health!

Going one step further, the consumption of alcohol, excess: caffeine, junk foods, processed refined foods, saturated and hydrogenated fats, (which means that a liquid oil has been processed into a solid form like margarine), salt, sugar, artificial sweeteners, and white flour are typically avoided in an anti-cancer diet.

Anti-cancer diets typically include living, raw, leafy, colorful, alkalizing, antioxidant-rich and enzyme-rich organic foods, with little meats or dairy, and typically limit dietary fat to 10-20% of total caloric intake.

Anti-cancer diets include an abundance of organic **fruits and vegetables** and may reduce the risk of breast cancer by 46%.[58, 59] Berries are typically high in anti-oxidants, which protect our cells from damage caused by the free-radicals that are created as our cells metabolize or encounter environmental pollution. For more information on anti-cancer diets, visit Ask Dr. Sears at www.askdrsears.com/html/4/T040300.asp.

Cruciferous vegetables are those with crowning heads like broccoli, cabbage, and cauliflower, and are particularly rich in anti-cancer nutrients, as are garlic, onions, red peppers, and tomatoes. In a Harvard survey, women who ate only one daily serving of a vitamin A rich food had 25% more breast cancer than those women who ate at least two servings a day. Dark, leafy greens, orange and yellow produce are good sources of vitamin A (beta–carotene), i.e. carrots.

Yet another healthy group of vegetables include legumes, which are plants with pods that contain seeds or beans. They often include enzymes and phytoestrogens that can help reduce estrogen levels in the breasts. **Enzymes** are critical for many bodily functions, including food digestion and ultimately, the body's ability to absorb nutrients. Without adequate enzymes, we become malnourished.

This can lead to degeneration, arthritis, heart disease, and cancer. Raw, living foods that are not overcooked provide enzymes. Cooking above 118°F typically destroys enzymes. Some foods release their enzymes when slightly cooked. For instance, slightly cooking carrots breaks down their tough cellular wall, and makes nutrients more available to the body.

Dry nuts, grains, seeds and legumes have built-in protection in the form of enzyme inhibitors. These inhibitors prevent enzymes from being activated until the seed is germinated, or sprouted. To activate their enzymes and make them bio-available, we need to sprout nuts, grains, seeds, and legumes. **Sprouting** involves soaking in water for 8 hours to 12 days. Sprouting books and charts available at many health food stores provide specifics and make this process easier.

Soy is an example of a legume known for its phytoestrogens. But it comes with good and bad aspects. That is, it is good in some forms and for some women, but not all forms and not for all women. Soy contains many phytonutrients and isoflavones, which are phytochemicals with potent antioxidant properties and many health benefits. However, to maintain the synergistic, or combined value, of these nutrients, consume soy in natural and whole-food forms of edamame, which is a whole, green soybean, tempeh, soy sprouts, tofu, and others.

Fermented forms of soy products contain probiotics, particularly the friendly bacteria lactobacilli, that ease digestion and have higher isoflavone availability. Fermented soy products include: natto, miso, tamari, tempeh, soy sauces, and fermented tofu and soymilks. Of course soy forms should be organic to avoid synthetic chemicals and organochlorines. Non GMO means the soybean is not a genetically modified organism.

This means that the potentially less ideal forms of soy include those that are not organic, have been genetically modified, overly processed, or refined, isolated, or concentrated. While research only recently began gathering data on the long-term effects of these forms, it has already been shown that some of these forms, particularly low-quality soy protein concentrates and isoflavone isolates can inhibit protein and mineral absorption. Inferior or low-quality products are often processed with chemicals and at high temperatures.

Now that we have covered different forms of soy, let's explain why soy isn't right for everyone. For some people, soy, especially in low-quality products, can cause allergic reactions, be hard to digest, and can reduce pancreatic enzymes. For these people, soy, particularly low-quality soy, is likely *not* the best choice.

Regarding women, soy can add to the estrogen activity in the breasts of women with low estrogen, or lower estrogen activity in the breasts of women with excess estrogen.

Here's an example. Imagine a row of seats in an auditorium or a stadium. Each seat represents an estrogen receptor site in the breasts. Now, imagine that a little girl sits in a seat. She is like a weak estrogen or phytoestrogen and now her seat, or space, is occupied. Next, imagine that a large muscular man approaches the little girl. While he is much stronger, he would not displace her from her seat. Instead, he passes by to find an available seat. He represents stronger estrogens in the body.

If there are unoccupied estrogen receptor sites in the breasts, they can become occupied by phytoestrogens and slightly add to the estrogen activity in women with low estrogen. However, for women with excess estrogen, some phytoestrogens actually compete with the stronger estrogens for receptor sites and can slightly reduce estrogen activity. In Chapter 8, we will reveal how certain breast thermography can help to indirectly assess the level of estrogen stimulation in the breasts.

Another dietary consideration includes fiber. Women whose diets are consistently high in **fiber** are expected to have less risk for breast cancer, as high fiber helps reduce estrogen levels. The American Cancer Society recommends 30 grams of fiber every day. Fiber binds with wastes, toxins, and estrogens in the intestines for elimination from the body.

You probably know that whole grains, oatmeal, beans, fruits, and vegetables provide fiber. Did you also know that quality psyllium husks and seeds can be an effective fiber supplement? Unlike supplements, however, fiber-rich whole foods provide additional nutrients as well. Don't forget: if you supplement your diet with fiber, be sure to increase your water intake, or you can become constipated. For more info on fiber, visit the Harvard School of Public Health at www.hsph.harvard.edu/nutritionsource/fiber. html.

Some researchers attribute up to 25% of all breast cancers to **dietary fats,** while others find no direct cause-and-effect relationship. Breast cancer risk is increased not so much by the amount of fat, but by the type of fat eaten. Most of us have heard the importance of eating monounsaturated fats rather than saturated fats.

Monounsaturated fats are typically liquid at room temperature, but solidify when refrigerated, while saturated fats are usually solid at room temperature. One Swedish study reported that monounsaturated fats, like those found in olive oil and canola oil, reduce the risk of breast cancer by 45%.[46]

Another study indicates that Greek women who eat **olive oil** more than once a day can reduce their risk of breast cancer by 25%.[58] On the island of Crete, which has some of the lowest rates of breast cancer in the world, women get up to 60% of their calories from fat.[28]   However, most U.S. prevention diets limit dietary fats to 20% of daily caloric intake. Our education group supports a low-percentage concept of 20-30%.

Look for organic, first cold-pressed, extra- virgin olive oils in containers that reduce sun exposure and heat, which can destroy essential fatty acids. Avoid using excess heat with oils, which can destroy essential fatty acids and create damaging free radicals. (Similarly, charred foods are actually cancer-causing, so avoiding the blackened portions of charbroiled foods is a healthy choice.)

Fats from non-organic sources of dairy, meats, oils, and nuts can contain large amounts of organochlorines. **Hydrogenated fats**, which are liquid oils processed into a solid form like those in most margarines and many packaged foods, contain trans-fatty acids which are cancer-causing. On the other hand, fats from organic olive oil and organic butter can reduce the risk of breast cancer because they contain some of the healthful phytochemicals that stop the initiation and progress of breast cancer.

Many researchers agree that 10-20% of daily caloric intake should be in the form of essential fatty acids, **EFAs,** referred to as **Omega-3s and 6s.**[60] (Omega 9s are synthe-sized in the body, so they are not considered essential.)

Current research indicates that the Omega 3s have therapeutic benefits in reducing high triglycerides, lowering hypertension, regulating irregular heart beat as well as assisting in learning disorders, infant brain development and menopausal discomforts. Some Omega 3s and 6s can aid in improving diabetic neuropathy, rheumatoid arthritis, PMS, skin disorders such as psoriasis and eczema, and cancer treatment.[61]

Fish and flax seed are rich in Omega-3s, while borage oil is rich in Omega-6s. (Evening primrose oil and black currant oil are other common forms of supplementation for Omega -6.)

COMMON SOURCES OF EFAs

Omega 3	Omega 6	Omega 9
black currant seed/oil	black currant seed/oil	almond/oil
canola oil	borage oil	avocado/oil
fish/oils	canola oil	butter
flax seed/oil	corn oil	cashew/oil
hemp seed/oil	evening primrose oil	filbert/oil
soybean/oil	flax seed/oil	hazelnut/oil
walnuts/oil	hemp seed/oil	land-animal fat
	pumpkin seed/oil	macadamia/oil
	safflower oil	olive/oil
	sesame oil	peanut/oil
	soybean/oil	pecan/oil
	sunflower seed/oil	pistachio/oil
	walnuts/oil	

The typical American diet is already rich in Omega 6s and can render Omega 6 to Omega 3 ratios of 20:1 to 50:1. While it is important to get both forms of essential fatty acids, **experts suggest adding Omega 3s to our diets while simultaneously reducing Omega 6s.**

Studies indicate that the risk of developing breast cancer decreases as the ratio of Omega 6 to Omega 3s approaches 1:1. Hence the need to add Omega 3s, which commonly involves flax and/or fish oil supplements. A natural form of vitamin E with mixed tocopherols and tocotrienols (groups of antioxidants) is a good complement to EFAs, and is good for breast health and cancer prevention.

Eating the right type and ratio of fats can be helpful in reducing the risk of breast cancer. For perspective and more information on the various forms of fats visit Ask Dr. Sears at www.askdrsears.com/html/4/T041300.asp, the Harvard School of Public Health at www.hsph.

harvard.edu/nutritionsource/fats.html, Women-to-Women
at www.womentowomen.com/LIBcholesterolandfat.asp,
and Udo Erasmus, author of *Fats that Heal Fats That Kill*, at
http://www.udoerasmus.com/FAQ.htm#1_1.
To help identify which oils to use at various cooking
temperatures, visit the Spectrum Organics charts at
www.spectrumorganics.com/index.php?id=182.

Have you heard about the glycemic index? It refers to how
fast a carbohydrate breaks down and how it effects blood
sugar levels. **High glycemic foods** elevate blood sugar and
insulin levels, stimulate fat-storage, worsen hyperactivity,
reduce sports performance and increase the risk of Type II
diabetes.

On the other hand, **low glycemic foods** help maintain
more stable blood sugar levels to reduce the food-craving
hormones which can cause chemically triggered cravings
for food and uncontrolled eating binges.

Research conducted through Harvard Medical School finds
that women with diabetes have 1.17 times greater risk of
developing breast cancer than women without diabetes.
However, risk increases only for post-menopausal women.
For more information on glycemic index and load lists,
visit the websites www.mendosa.com and
www.glycemicindex.com.

We have all heard that we should get our **vitamins and
minerals**. But did you know that most vitamins cannot do
their jobs in our bodies without minerals? Or, that in 1936,
U.S. Senate Document 264 announced that our farm soils
were severely depleted of minerals? The 1992 Earth
Summit Report delivered similar findings.

While farmers typically supplement with three minerals, namely phosphorous, nitrogen, and potassium, we humans need over 70 different minerals everyday. When our diet is void of these minerals, we can develop cravings, binge eat, develop obesity, and still be malnourished.

Do you know that the U.S. Department of Agriculture recommends 9 servings of fruits and vegetables a day for active males and reports that less than 1% of children under age 16 get 5 servings a day? The general consensus among the health industry is that **Americans need to eat more fresh fruits and vegetables on a daily basis**.

Because so many of us do not eat enough of the foods that we need for proper nutrition, the American Medical Association suggests that doctors recommend **nutritional supplementation**.[62]

This should include a full spectrum of nutrients in the right form and proportions for each of us, including vitamins, minerals, essential fatty acids, and perhaps enzymes, probiotics, and more. Again, please consult with a qualified healthcare provider regarding your individual supplementation needs. Keep in mind that supplements are intended to supplement a good diet, not replace it.

Some health food stores provide **clinical nutritionists** for (complimentary) consultations with customers, like Lisa High, profiled in the chapter, "About the Authors". Her specialties in nutrition include supplementation, blood sugar and weight management, food allergies, and cardiovascular support. Consult your local health food store for access to Certified Clinical Nutritionists or Registered Dietitians or ask your healthcare provider for a referral to a qualified nutritionist in your area.

Here are two more tips for maintaining more of the nutritional value in food. First, **cook foods appropriately**. Some foods require low and gentle heat, some are best prepared by steaming, and some are most nutritious in their raw form. For example, below are the effects of boiling broccoli on some if its nutrients:

Broccoli

	Units	Raw	Boiled	% Change
Key Minerals				
Calcium	mg	47	40	- 15%
Iron	mg	0.73	0.67	- 8%
Magnesium	mg	21	21	- 0%
Potassium	mg	316	293	- 7%
Key Vitamins				
A	mcg	31	98	+ 216 %
C	mg	89	42	- 53%
E	mg	0.78	1.45	+ 86%
K	mcg	102	141	+ 39%

Source: U.S. Department of Agriculture National Nutrition Database for Standard Reference, Release 18 (2005), NDB Nos. 11090, 11742.

For more information on how cooking methods impact nutrients, visit the U.S. Department of Agriculture's Table of Nutrient Retention Factors, at www.nal.usda.gov/fnic/ foodcomp/Data/, or consult with nutritionists, professional chefs, or the food preparation books available in most health food stores.

Second, since **microwaves** disturb the molecular bonds of foods, some people choose to minimize their use, and instead, use more stovetops and ovens.

For more information on the potential implications of microwaved foods on our health, visit the Global Healing Center at www.ghchealth.com/microwave-ovens-the-proven-dangers.html and www.buergerwelle.de/pdf/microwave_cooking.pdf.

PART THREE

RISK ASSESSMENT & MONITORING/THERMAL IMAGING

8

Assessing the Collective Effect of All Risk Factors on Breast Health

Now that you have a better understanding of how genetics, estrogen, the environment, health, lifestyle and diet can impact your breast health, you may be ready to address multiple risk factors.

At this point you may be thinking that there are so many factors that impact breast health that you are not sure where to begin. If you have completed your Better Breast Health – *for Life!*™ Workshop and Worksheet, however, you have identified which risk factors apply to you, and understand the relative significance of each.

Now you can prioritize only those risk factors that pertain to you and focus on *your* highest priorities, taking action to potentially reduce the effect of each on your breast health.

There remains one additional question, **"What is the collective effect of all these factors on my breast health today?"**

Knowing the answer to this question is another important step in a proactive prevention process. For example, if a woman learns that the collective effect of all these risk factors on her breast health is favorable, then she will have less concern or motivation for change. However, a woman who learns that her collective effect is not favorable is more likely to be motivated to address more of these risk factors. While a favorable outcome may be encouraging, a less than favorable outcome may motivate a woman to take steps that may preempt or prevent breast cancer in the future.

There is a test available to help answer this question. The test involves **thermal breast imaging**. You may have heard it's old name referred to as **thermography**, but today's technology has the capability to more accurately assess the effects of these risk factors and, in particular, estrogen activity.

Let's explain how this new test works with some background information.

At a cellular level, active cancer cells seek their own blood supply for nourishment. They support their own growth by secreting chemicals like nitric oxide into the surrounding tissue in order to dilate, or expand, the blood vessels there to deliver more blood. This process is referred to as **vasodilation**.[63, 64]

They also create new blood vessels to route blood from our circulation system directly to themselves. This process is referred to as **neoangiogenesis**. These newly formed blood vessels typically form dilated looping patterns around the active cancer.[65] At this point the active cancer cells have a continuous supply of nutrients and can multiply and grow more quickly. At this point, the cancer is considered **metabolically active**.

The average active cancer typically doubles in size every three months, while the aggressive active cancer typically doubles in size every 6-8 weeks. (The most aggressive cancers can double in size in as few as 8 days.)[66] While today's mammography is enabling the detection of smaller cancers, cancer has typically grown for 3 to10 years before diagnosis.

This is why someone exposed to a risk factor may not know that cancer has initiated – because it can take up to 10 years for the cancer to grow large enough to be detected.

Research suggests that when active cancer cells occupy a space as small as 1/5 of 1mm, or about the size of the tip of a ball point pen, they begin to develop their own blood supply.[67] While this is too small for detection by palpation, it is the subject of thermal breast imaging. By looking for signs of a developing blood supply, thermal breast imaging assesses the *risk* of developing cancer.

However, it is not a diagnostic test. It is **a risk marker test**, providing biological risk indication and assessment, like the BRCA-1 and BRCA-2 breast cancer gene tests. (Some thermal breast imagers provide no risk evaluation with their service, and may be perceived as providing a "detection" service – an alternative to a mammogram. Unfortunately, this misconception adds to the decades-old, faulty notion that a thermogram can replace a mammogram.)

Thermography is approved by the U.S. Food and Drug Administration (FDA) as an adjunctive, or complementary test to mammography, like ultrasounds and MRIs. Thermal imaging can add to the findings of mammograms and assess the risk of developing cancer. While it is not yet broadly available and not many doctors are familiar with it, demand for this test will increase its availability and awareness among doctors.

Since the thermal imaging industry currently works without enforced standards, quality and output across providers can vary greatly. When looking for a service provider near you, consider whether or not the service includes **thermobiological, or TH, risk ratings and estrogen stimulation assessment with black and white images**. Let's use The Thermogram Center in Colorado as an example.

In addition to detailed explanation, the center uses thermobiological risk ratings, on a scale of 1 to 5, to assess the risk of developing breast cancer in each breast. While these risk ratings were established decades ago by researchers of thermography, subsequent studies continue to support their validity as a risk indicator. [68]

For instance, long-term follow-up findings reported in *Cancer* and *BioMedical Thermology* indicate that 40% of patients with high and highest risk, TH 4 or TH 5 ratings, are diagnosed with breast cancer within 10 years, with the majority being diagnosed in the first 5 years. [69,70] In addition, a study conducted at Northwestern University's Department of Obstetrics and Gynecology reports that abnormal thermal exams are ten times as significant a risk factor as is family history. [42]

So, while a TH 2 indicates low risk and may suggest that a patient live a healthy lifestyle, a TH 5 indicates highest risk and warrants further evaluation by a breast specialist to determine if there is a sizable cancerous tumor.

While 7 to 9 views of the breasts are captured in black and white and in color at the Center, the following chest views, usually shown in color, are shown on the following page in grayscale.

Thermobiological Risk Ratings

TH1 — *Lowest Risk*

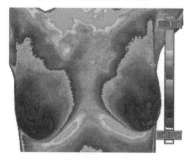

TH2 — *Low Risk*

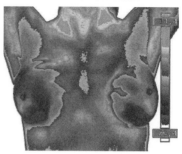

Level of Response:

- 12 month thermal imaging follow-up for women over 30 years of age
- examinations directed by the patient's physician
- live a healthy lifestyle

TH3 — *Medium Risk*

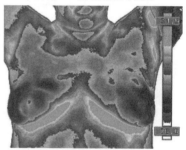

Level of Response:

- 6 month thermal imaging follow-up
- examinations directed by the patient's physician, i.e. correlation by mammogram or ultrasound
- manage risk factors: estrogenic, health & lifestyle, diet, environmental

TH4 — *High Risk*

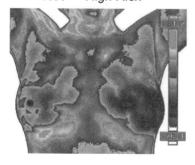

TH5 — *Highest Risk*

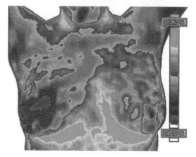

Level of Response:

- examinations directed by the patient's physician, i.e. follow-up by mammogram, ultrasound, and/or MRI
- 3 month thermal imaging follow-up if no sizable tumor is detected
- optimize risk factors: estrogenic, health & lifestyle, diet, environmental

If a sizable cancerous tumor is revealed upon further evaluation, then thermal imaging has supported early detection. If not, then the patient can address those risk factors for which she has some control to potentially impact and reduce her overall breast cancer risk. Thermal imaging can also be used to **help monitor the effects of prevention or treatment** on breast cancer risk over time – to see if the steps being taken are working to reduce a woman's risk.

For example, the following individual added certified lymphatic massage therapy to her prevention efforts. While there is no proof of a direct cause and effect, her thermal images suggest improvement: her right breast risk rating decreased from a TH 4 to a TH 2+. (Again, these images typically appear in color, not grayscale.)

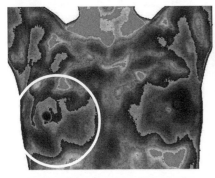 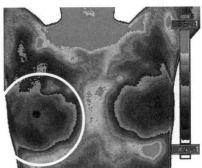

R: TH 4, L: TH 2   R: TH 2+, L: TH 2

Of course, some patients do not improve:

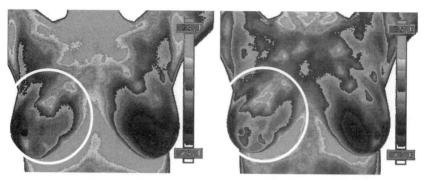

R: TH 4, L: TH 1   R: TH 4+, L: TH 1

This patient's right breast risk rating did not improve, prompting her to take further action.

Additionally, the Center provides black and white images of the vascularity of the breasts and grades the level of vascular dilation seen, relative to a state of lactation, when estrogen levels are high. The resulting **Vascular Display Grades,** which indiretly assess the level of estrogen stimulation, are shown on the following page on a scale of 1 to 4.

This is important because, according to the National Institutes of Health, our breasts can hold 10 to 50 times more estrogen than a blood test may reveal… and as we have discussed, prolonged exposure to excess estrogen is the highest known risk factor for breast cancer. With the latest thermal imaging, women have another way of monitoring (albeit indirectly) the estrogen activity in their breasts, not just in their blood, urine, or saliva. (Since there are many factors that can contribute to increased blood flow to the breasts, it is important that thermal findings be correlated with the patient's particular situation by a qualified health provider.)

Vascular Display Grades

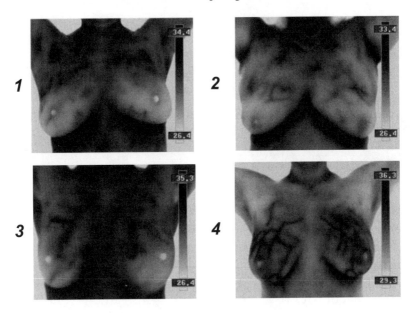

Grade 1 is commonly seen in postmenopausal women, while Grade 2 is commonly seen between puberty and menopause. Grade 3 is commonly seen with HRT, birth control pill use, progesterone deficiency, and large breast size. Grade 4 is commonly seen in lactation, pregnancy, and exogenous estrogen usage.

Black and white images also enhance the ability to study the vascularity and blood supply in the breasts. For the following individual, further evaluation rendered a diagnosis of cancer of the left breast, pictured on the right of each of her chest views. Note the extensive blood supply in the left breast, which elevated surface temperatures in excess of 6°C when compared to the right breast.

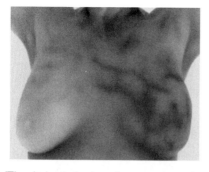

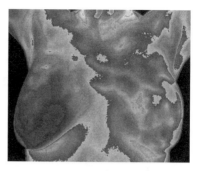

(The darkest shades of gray represent the highest temperatures)

(The lightest shades of gray represent higher temperatures)

Below is an example of a patient whose higher-than-expected Vascular Display Grade (VDG) prompted intervention. After a 3 month nutritionally-based regimen to support estrogen metabolism, her VDG decreased from a 3 to a 1, demonstrating that while exposure to excess estrogen may be a significant risk factor, she was able to reduce it relatively easily:

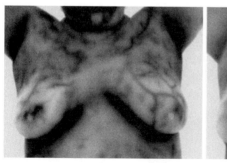

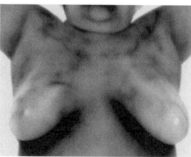

VDG 3   VDG 1

For more information on thermobiological risk ratings and Vascular Display Grades with thermal breast imaging examples **in color**, visit The Thermogram Center website www.thermogramcenter.com.

In summary, today's thermal breast imaging can support prevention, intervention, and early detection. It can be an integral part of every woman's proactive prevention journey, given that it can help to monitor the results of her efforts.

> "I like to think of my thermal breast imaging as a way of understanding how all the risk factors are impacting my breast health at any given point in time. If I don't like the results, I make changes in one or more of these factors and monitor the impact with a new risk assessment. It is empowering me on my journey towards better breast health."
>
> — Tina

PART FOUR

SUMMARY &
SUPPLEMENTAL
INFORMATION

9

Summary

We trust that after completing this material you have a greater sense of control over risk factors in your life and feel empowered with knowledge on ways to potentially reduce them.

In summary… to support good breast health, **complete your Better Breast Health -** *for Life!*™ **Workshop and Risk Factors Worksheet,** and learn if there is a thermal breast imaging provider in your area to **get your thermal imaging risk assessment** with thermobiological risk ratings and estrogen assessment.

Then, take appropriate levels of action. Remember the saying, **"an ounce of prevention is worth a pound of cure…"** This applies to *all* levels of risk, not just *high* levels of risk. Use the **"Actions Checklist"** document from the CD to record and track the action steps you intend to take on your journey to better breast health. This checklist is shown on page 70.

Consult with qualified healthcare providers along your journey.

For more information on breast health seminars at your workplace, organization, or institution, please contact us at info@BetterBreastHealthforLife.com or at 866-492-2174.

Finally, please share this information with anyone you care about, as the risk factors that contribute to breast cancer are often associated with other forms of cancer, in men and women alike.

Actions Checklist - check the box that corresponds to your intended action steps.

To Begin	☐	complete the Better Breast Health - *for Life!* ™ Workshop and Risk Factors Worksheet
	☐	acquire initial thermal imaging risk assessment with estrogen evaluation
Genetics & Estrogen	☐	obtain qualified health provider(s) for consultation
	☐	reshape body to approach a waist to hip ratio less than .81
	☐	reduce weight to approach a Body Mass Index under 25
	☐	maintain hormones in proper balance
	☐	maintain healthy estrogen metabolism
Environment	☐	obtain qualified health provider(s) for consultation
	☐	reduce/limit toxin or carcinogen exposure, i.e agricultural and petro-chemicals
	☐	focus on hormone-free, chemical-free organic meats, dairy, and produce
	☐	drink 1/2 to 1 ounce of *pure* water per pound of body weight each day
	☐	reduce/limit pollutant or chemical exposure, i.e. non-natural personal products
	☐	use proper plastics when glass, ceramics, or stainless steel aren't an option
	☐	avoid radiation exposure to breasts if age 8-20 years old
	☐	reduce/limit high-powered EMF (electromagmetic frequency) exposure
	☐	reduce exposure to household EMF by staying 28" away from electric sources
Health & Lifestyle	☐	obtain qualified health provider(s) for consultation
	☐	maintain regular sleep patterns and proper melatonin levels
	☐	reduce smoking of tobacco
	☐	reduce alcohol consumption and/or support it with a liver-supporting regimen
	☐	drink 1/2 to 1 ounce of *pure* water per pound of body weight each day
	☐	acquire sufficient sunlight and maintain proper vitamin D levels
	☐	resolve deep, long-lasting emotional trauma/stress and grief
	☐	reduce/resolve daily stress levels
	☐	wear bras that are professionally "fitted" to the breasts
	☐	support lymph fluid circulation
	☐	maintain moderate exercise levels
	☐	cleanse bodily systems, i.e. colon, liver, lymph
	☐	reduce chronic inflammation
	☐	address opportunities to reduce or complement medication or drug use
	☐	address mercury or heavy metal issues
	☐	maintain proper iodine levels and thyroid function
Diet	☐	obtain qualified health provider(s) for consultation
	☐	focus on hormone-free, chemical-free organic meats, dairy, and produce
	☐	maintain healthy alkaline and acidic food proportions
	☐	increase servings of fresh fruits and vegetables, approaching 9 servings a day
	☐	focus on eating more raw and/or gently cooked foods for their enzyme value
	☐	eat more sprouted nuts, grains, and seeds
	☐	eat only high-quality, organic and natural whole-food sources of soy
	☐	maintain adequate levels of friendly bacteria in the intestines
	☐	maintain adequate fiber intake, near 30g per day
	☐	focus on eating more organic, monounsaturated fats than any other forms of fats
	☐	approach an Omega 6:Omega 3 ratio towards 1:1
	☐	maintain a diet resulting in healthy glycemic values and loads
	☐	maintain adequate daily nutritional supplementation
	☐	employ optimal cooking methods
Monitor Your Results	☐	monitor the effects of your actions with sequential thermal imaging
		- is each breast's risk rating improving?
		- what is the level of estrogen stimulation?
	☐	consult and strategize with your qualified healthcare provider(s) regarding additional opportunities to support your journey towards better breast health

10

Lessons in Breast Care... Lessons for Life!

By Glenna Biehler and Tirza Derflinger

My name is Glenna, and life seemed to be getting back to normal after the birth of my third child in October 2004. Following a difficult pregnancy that included three months of bed rest, my husband and I, decided that our family was now complete and we were looking forward to the many wonderful life experiences that would accompany a family of five. Little did we know that one month after our daughter was born I would find a lump in my left breast.

The symptoms and timing led my doctor and me to believe it was a simple case of mastitis, an infection in the milk duct. My doctor prescribed an antibiotic and told me she would do a thorough examination at my six week check-up. We enjoyed Thanksgiving with our families not knowing that within two weeks our world would be turned inside-out.

When my doctor performed a palpable breast exam, she determined that it was not a clogged milk duct like we had first thought. She sent me directly to radiology for an ultrasound to determine if it was a fluid mass or solid mass. The test showed a solid mass meaning I would have to have a biopsy. My husband and I were still not overly alarmed since I was only 37 years old, had no family history of breast cancer, didn't smoke, ate a healthy diet, and exercised regularly. Unfortunately, I would find out that such behaviors don't always guarantee that our bodies won't develop problems.

On December 10, I received the horrible news that I had been diagnosed with breast cancer. Many thoughts went through my head, most of them involving my husband and three small children. I couldn't fathom how this had happened to me. Two days later, life was no longer in my control. I had two surgeries, many doctor appointments and lots of difficult decisions to make about what treatment was best suited for my situation.

On January 3, 2005 when most people are excited and looking forward to a new year, I was starting my long journey with chemotherapy. I would go on to do four months of chemotherapy followed by six weeks of radiation. It was a long road of sickness dealing with chemotherapy and the drugs that were used to combat the many side effects.

Shortly after I began my treatment I would have trouble sleeping because of the steroids that were used in my regimen. On one of these late nights while lying in bed debating with myself and God about this horrific change in my life I decided that I needed to find a way to turn this unthinkable negative into a positive that could help other women in the future. This is when the idea for a breast awareness campaign targeting pregnant and nursing mothers came to me.

I had always been vigilant in performing monthly breast exams but became remiss during my pregnancies. I believe this is common among many women and I'm determined to convey a message to all women that we need to be aware of our changing bodies - and our breasts - during this special time. As a result, I now offer breast awareness posters, shown below, especially for OB-GYN office waiting rooms.

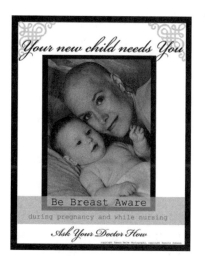

The intent of the poster is to move women in such a way that they will ask about breast exams during this ever-important time. Ultimately, I seek the support of a health organization to employ the image on informational brochures for expectant mothers.

Glenna's story is one of many personally moving stories that I hear. My name is Tirza and I am a breast imaging technician at The Thermogram Center, TTC. Since opening in 2002, the center has been moved by its own trials and tribulations experienced on its journey to introduce the latest breast test, thermal imaging, formerly thermography, into patient care.

While women embrace the test, already FDA-approved, the AMA awaits the establishment of the protocols that direct doctors' care once a patient's breast cancer risk has been assessed with thermal imaging. This step is certainly necessary for broad-scale integration into patient care, and part of the huge responsibility of the AMA. Until the test is standard-of-care, the struggle to gain acceptance among the medical field is a daunting task, and for good reason.

In the beginning, I thought thermal imaging might be the "magic bullet"… a test so sensitive, that it could exceed the capability of mammograms. But then it finally happened: in our fourth year of service, the first reported false negative appeared. Julie, a TTC patient who had a normal mammogram and a normal thermogram, became diagnosed with breast cancer. Both breast exams missed signs consistent with cancer. Stunned, we asked, "How could this happen?"

Not being a cancer doctor, I have much to learn about the cancer process. Like many women, I want to believe that there can be one test that can "see" cancer at a very early stage. Unfortunately, this is not the case – and may never be. And for Julie, thermal imaging is clearly NOT a magic bullet.

Thermal imaging's inherent strength lies in its ability to see signs of the developing blood supply that cancer cells create for themselves. But this only happens with active cancers. The more aggressive the cancer, the more obvious the signs of a developing blood supply. But what about the less active cancers that are slow-growing or in-situ? (In-situ cancers have not spread to surrounding breast tissue.)

These types of cancer are less likely to have formed their own blood supply and less likely to be visible in thermograms. In these cases, mammograms and/or ultrasounds are more likely to detect the cancer. Julie's cancer was an in-situ cancer of the duct that recently activated to invade surrounding tissue. Fortunately, she felt pain that prompted the ultrasound and MRI that led to her early diagnosis.

There are two important lessons in these stories that can benefit women. First, it is important to be breast-aware at every life stage, whether under age 40 (when cancers are most aggressive), pregnant or nursing (when tests are less sensitive), or over age 50 (when most breast cancers are diagnosed). Second, it is important to understand each breast test's unique and complementary role in detection, and to employ any/all tests available in order to increase the likelihood of early detection. It's up to us women to be breast-aware and seek these tests to ensure potentially life-saving early detection. A reference table follows:

Breast Test	Palpation/Self-Exam	Thermogram	Mammogram	Ultrasound	MRI
Age Guidelines	20+	20+	40+	when warranted	when warranted
What it Detects	tissue changes	signs of active, aggressive cancer	masses, calcifications	fluid vs solid characteristics	extent and locations of cancer
Strengths	frequency, i.e monthly	signs of increased risk can prompt further evaluation, intervention & prevention efforts	standard test/universally understood; early detection possible	can help distinguish cancerous from non-cancerous masses, i.e. fibrocystic changes	can increase sensitivity of breast testing
Weaknesses	can be limited when breasts are dense or thick, or when lesion is deep	cannot precisely locate masses	can be limited when breast tissue is dense	can be limited when breast is fatty or thick	can be limited for in-situ cancer in the duct; expensive
What it means for women...	Women can participate in their breast evaluation process; complements all other breast exams	Good for: assessing risk of developing cancer; dense or thick tissue; pregnant/nursing mothers; complements all other breast exams	Good for: detecting lesions too deep to be palpable; seeing calcifications that may indicate in-situ cancer in the duct	Good for: dense tissue; evaluating a palpable mass or abnormal mammographic finding	Good: prior to surgery planning for known cancer; for high risk patients
Cost	low	moderate	moderate	moderate	high

For information on Glenna's campaign and poster purchases, e-mail glennabiehler@msn.com.

For information on thermal breast imaging, visit www.thermogramcenter.com or e-mail info@thermogramcenter.com.

For information on self-exams, mammograms, and ultrasound, visit www.cancer.org.

11

About the Authors

Below are the breast health specialists associated with the Breast Health Education Group, whose purpose is to educate women on the risk factors that contribute to the development of breast cancer. Because of their diverse specialties and backgrounds, each makes a valued and unique contribution.

Their specialties are often sought by women along their journey to better breast health. Each is profiled here so that you may familiarize yourself with the kinds of specialists that you may choose to seek in your local area.

Deborah Breakell, FNP at Helios Integrated Medicine: Deborah works with Pierre Brunschwig, MD. Deborah helps women make informed decisions about natural hormone therapy such as the use of progesterone, estriol, phytochemicals like diindolylmethane/Indole-3- carbinol , and phytoestrogens. They provide not only the Estronex test to assess the ratio of good to bad estrogen metabolites, but also provide saliva and/or serum testing for ovarian and adrenal hormones. To evaluate the body's immune system, they also provide a test called Elisa/ACT LRA that checks for heavy metals, antigens, environmental toxins, and other items. These tests help determine what needs to be detoxified from the body, what lifestyle changes may be needed, and how to support the body with nutrition. For more information, visit www.wellcast.org and www.helioshealthcenter.com.

Carrie Louise Daenell, ND: A graduate of Bastyr University, Dr. Daenell is a Naturopathic Doctor, a licensed primary care physician and an expert in the use of natural medicine. She specializes in bio-identical hormone replacement therapy, and healthy estrogen metabolism for women facing hormonal changes. She works closely with the Thermogram Center in order to help women correct any issues found during their breast imaging process, before they become serious health problems. Previously the managing editor of the Journal of Naturopathic Medicine, a director for the American Association of Naturopathic Physicians and the president of the Colorado Association of Naturopathic Physicians, she is currently writing a book on estrogen health and she practices in Denver, Co. For more information, visit www.DrDaenell.com.

Carol Dalton, NP at Helios Integrated Medicine: For over 35 years Carol has blended self-care alternative methods of testing and treatment with traditional medical approaches assisting patients in developing their own personal plans for optimal health. She sees patients in person at her Boulder office and has a large national practice with phone consultations. Tests and treatments for maintaining healthy breasts and treatment for various imbalances of breast health are an integral part of her care. During menopause she offers each woman options for individualized natural bio-identical HRT and other ways of supporting their health during this transition. Carol has produced over 30 audiocassette tapes on a variety of health issues and a video "Menopause: The Positive Change." For more information , visit www.women-health.com and www.helioshealthcenter.com.

John R.M. Day, MD, ABHM at Haelan LifeStream: Formerly a general surgeon in Boulder for 20 years, Dr. Day worked with breast cancer patients on a daily basis. He now works as a board-certified holistic practitioner, providing counseling for body, mind, emotions, and spirit. Other services include bio-identical hormone replacement therapy (BHRT), as well as bioenergy treatment. The Haelan LifeStream model is based on evolving the development of nutrition, exercise, mental and emotional clarity, self love, spiritual awareness/alignment, and vision work. Emphasis is given to resolving the remains of old emotional and physical trauma through cognitive awareness, trauma renegotiation, psych-k therapy, and bio-energy treatment. The model is appropriate for any person who seeks deeper levels of health and fulfillment in their life experience. Dr. Day practices in Boulder, CO. For more information, visit www.haelanlifestream.com.

Tirza Derflinger CTT, MBA-MOT at The Thermogram Center: Formerly a Medical Laboratory Specialist for the U.S. Army, Tirza is now President of The Thermogram Center, founder of the Breast Health Education Group, and lead author of Better Breast Health – *for Life!*™ At The Thermogram Center, Ms. Derflinger works with patients and their doctors to provide thermal imaging that monitors a woman's risk for developing breast cancer and assesses her level of estrogen stimulation, a known risk factor for breast cancer. Thermal imaging is being used to assess pain conditions and other health concerns, and to monitor the effects of treatment and preventive therapies on breast cancer risk. For more information, visit www.thermogramcenter.com.

Lisa High, MS, RD at Essential Nutrition: Lisa High is a Registered Dietitian. She holds a Bachelor of Science degree in Nutrition and Food Management and a Master of Science degree in Gerontology, the study of aging, Physiology, and Nutrition. She has studied nutrition and counseled clients on diet and health for nearly 10 years. Six of these years were spent at the world- renown Canyon Ranch Health Resort in Tucson, Arizona. She is the Nutrition Director of the Shape Your Life program, as seen in Shape Magazine, and is co-author of the Bone and Joint Health chapter in the upcoming "Nutrition and Alternative Medicine" textbook (CRC Press, to be released in 2005). She is a firm believer in the study and practice of natural medicine and studies the principles of Functional Medicine. For more information, visit www.eatwellfeelgood.com.

Kelly McAleese, MD at Women's Imaging Center: Dr. McAleese is a Diagnostic Radiologist with specialization in Women's Imaging. She is the Medical Director of the Women's Imaging Center in Denver, Co. that provides comprehensive, state-of-the-art imaging with a hands-on approach to patient care. Dr. McAleese understands the concepts of thermal breast imaging and uses its findings to direct her ultrasound examinations, and sometimes even biopsies. She lectures yearly at the Radiologic Society of North America (the largest medical meeting in the world) and anticipates the future of breast imaging may include mammography, ultrasound, MRI, and thermal imaging to enable earlier breast cancer detection. Dr. McAleese is an advocate for all women's health issues.

12

References & Resources

Audio Workshop CD, Risk Factors Worksheet & Actions Checklist

This publication includes a one-hour audio workshop CD, a Risk Factors Worksheet, and an Actions Checklist. With these, you can **attend our Better Breast Health -** *for Life!*™ **Workshop – without leaving home**!

We encourage you to complete the workshop and "Risk Factors Worksheet" before reviewing the book. Doing so will enable you **to identify and prioritize the risk factors present in** *your* **life**. Then you can focus on *your* highest priorities, learning how to impact them by referring to the contents of this book. Afterwards, you can use the "Actions Checklist" to record and track the action steps you have selected for yourself.

To listen to the audio CD, simply insert your CD into any CD player. To obtain a full-size (8.5"x11") worksheets, insert the CD into your computer CD driver and use your file directory software and printer to open and print the "Risk Factors Worksheet" shown on page 82 and the "Actions Checklist" shown on page 83.

This worksheet is intended to be used with the Better Breast Health - *for Life!*™ Audio Workshop CD and is designed to help you identify and prioritize areas of opportunity to reduce risk.

Areas of Opportunity & Risk Factors for Which Women Have Some Control (in the order each appears in the book, Better Breast Health - *for Life!*™)	Level of Added Risk
Prolonged or Continuous:	
waist to hip ratio greater than .81	H
Body Mass Index over 25	L to M
* no full-term pregnancy	L
* using HRT or estrogen useage now and have been for at least 5 years	L
* used birth control pills for at least 5 years prior to first full term pregnancy	M to H
* premature delivery before 32 weeks	L
* termination of teenage pregnancy between weeks 9 and 24	EH
improper estrogen metabolism or estrogen dominance	L
toxin or carcinogen exposure, i.e agricultural and petro-chemicals	H
pollutant or chemical exposure, i.e. non-natural personal or home cleaning products	L to M
radiation exposure to breasts aged 8-20 years old	L to M
high-powered EMF (electromagmetic frequency) exposure	EH
irregular sleep patterns	L to M
smoking of tobacco	L to M
alcohol consumption of at least 10 drinks/week	L to M
drink only small amount of pure water daily (far less than 1/2 oz/lb of body weight)	N
lack of sufficient sunlight	L
deep, long-lasting emotional trauma/stress	N
low to moderate daily stress levels	L
high daily stress levels	M
wearing bras more than 12 hrs/day, everyday, particularly if not professionally "fitted"	M
sedentary lifestyle with little or no exercise	L to M
never cleanse bodily systems	N
symptoms of chronic inflammation	L
medication or drug use	L to M
low iodine/underactive thyroid	L to M
diet is not organic or hormone free	N
acidic diet vs alkaline diet	N
cooked/refined diet vs raw diet	L
low fiber diet, i.e. less than 30g per day	L
majority of fat intake is not in the form of organic monounsaturated fats	L
Omega 6:Omega 3 ratio approaching 20+:1	L
diabetic or high glycemic (sugar/starch) diet and postmenopausal	L
little or no nutritional supplementation	N
microwaving as primary method of cooking	N

Row groups (left margin): Genetics & Estrogen; Environment; Health & Lifestyle; Diet.

N** = no clinical risk   L = Low; = 2X   M = Medium; > 2X and = 5X
H = High: > 5X and = 10X   EH = Extremely High; > 10X

* These items represent typical lifetime events rather than prolonged or continuous situations.
** These items represent potential areas of opportunity to support good health, but have no clinically-established association with the development of breast cancer. These areas may be investigated in the future for their association with the development of breast cancer and added risk.

		Actions Checklist - check the box that corresponds to your intended action steps.

To Begin	☐	complete the Better Breast Health - *for Life!* ™ Workshop and Risk Factors Worksheet
	☐	acquire initial thermal imaging risk assessment with estrogen evaluation
Genetics & Estrogen	☐	obtain qualified health provider(s) for consultation
	☐	reshape body to approach a waist to hip ratio less than .81
	☐	reduce weight to approach a Body Mass Index under 25
	☐	maintain hormones in proper balance
	☐	maintain healthy estrogen metabolism
Environment	☐	obtain qualified health provider(s) for consultation
	☐	reduce/limit toxin or carcinogen exposure, i.e agricultural and petro-chemicals
	☐	focus on hormone-free, chemical-free organic meats, dairy, and produce
	☐	drink 1/2 to 1 ounce of *pure* water per pound of body weight each day
	☐	reduce/limit pollutant or chemical exposure, i.e. non-natural personal products
	☐	use proper plastics when glass, ceramics, or stainless steel aren't an option
	☐	avoid radiation exposure to breasts if age 8-20 years old
	☐	reduce/limit high-powered EMF (electromagmetic frequency) exposure
	☐	reduce exposure to household EMF by staying 28" away from electric sources
Health & Lifestyle	☐	obtain qualified health provider(s) for consultation
	☐	maintain regular sleep patterns and proper melatonin levels
	☐	reduce smoking of tobacco
	☐	reduce alcohol consumption and/or support it with a liver-supporting regimen
	☐	drink 1/2 to 1 ounce of *pure* water per pound of body weight each day
	☐	acquire sufficient sunlight and maintain proper vitamin D levels
	☐	resolve deep, long-lasting emotional trauma/stress and grief
	☐	reduce/resolve daily stress levels
	☐	wear bras that are professionally "fitted" to the breasts
	☐	support lymph fluid circulation
	☐	maintain moderate exercise levels
	☐	cleanse bodily systems, i.e. colon, liver, lymph
	☐	reduce chronic inflammation
	☐	address opportunities to reduce or complement medication or drug use
	☐	address mercury or heavy metal issues
	☐	maintain proper iodine levels and thyroid function
Diet	☐	obtain qualified health provider(s) for consultation
	☐	focus on hormone-free, chemical-free organic meats, dairy, and produce
	☐	maintain healthy alkaline and acidic food proportions
	☐	increase servings of fresh fruits and vegetables, approaching 9 servings a day
	☐	focus on eating more raw and/or gently cooked foods for their enzyme value
	☐	eat more sprouted nuts, grains, and seeds
	☐	eat only high-quality, organic and natural whole-food sources of soy
	☐	maintain adequate levels of friendly bacteria in the intestines
	☐	maintain adequate fiber intake, near 30g per day
	☐	focus on eating more organic, monounsaturated fats than any other forms of fats
	☐	approach an Omega 6:Omega 3 ratio towards 1:1
	☐	maintain a diet resulting in healthy glycemic values and loads
	☐	maintain adequate daily nutritional supplementation
	☐	employ optimal cooking methods
Monitor Your Results	☐	monitor the effects of your actions with sequential thermal imaging - is each breast's risk rating improving? - what is the level of estrogen stimulation?
	☐	consult and strategize with your qualified healthcare provider(s) regarding additional opportunities to support your journey towards better breast health

A quick-reference alkaline/acidic food chart is provided below:

Common Acid Categories		Common Alkaline Categories
Alcohol	Nuts, Most	Flours (buckwheat and millet)
Coffees	Poultry	Fruits, Most
Dairy, Most	Soda/Soft Drinks	Nuts, Some
Fish, All	Sugars	Sprouted Nuts & Seeds
Flours, Most	Overcooked Foods, All	Vegetables, Most
Meats, All	Unsprouted Nuts & Seeds	

Common Acid Foods

Bacon	Olives
Beans	Organ Meats
Beef	Oysters
Bran, Wheat	Peanut Butter
Bran, Oats	Peanuts
Bread, White	Peas, Dried
Bread, Wheat	Poultry
Carob	Plums
Catsup	Pork
Cheese	Prunes
Chicken	Refined Sugar
Cocoa	Salmon
Coffee	Sardines
Cod Fish	Sausage
Corn Starch	Scallops
Corn Oil	Shrimp
Corn Syrup	Soft drinks
Coconut	Sugar
Corned Beef	Squash, Winter
Crackers, Soda	Sunflower Seeds
Cranberries	Tea
Currants	Turkey
Eggs	Veal
Fish	Vegetable Oil
Flour, White	Walnuts
Flour, Wheat	Water, Tap
Haddock	Wheat Germ
Ice Cream	Yogurt
Lamb	
Legumes	**Better Acid Foods**
Lobster	Barley
Milk, Cow	Blueberries
Meat	Corn
Mustard	Honey
Nuts, Most	Lentils, Dried

Oatmeal
Olive Oil
Pasta
Rice, all

Neutral Foods

Butter
Water, Distilled

Alkaline Foods

Almonds	Grapes
Amaranth	Green Beans
Apples	Green Peas
Apricots	Lemons
Avocados	Lettuce
Bananas	Lima Beans, Dried
Beet Greens	Lima Beans, Green
Beets	Limes
Buckwheat	Milk, Goat
Buckwheat Flour	Millet
Blackberries	Millet Flour
Broccoli	Molasses
Brussel Sprouts	Mushrooms
Brazil Nuts	Onions
Cabbage	Oranges
Cantalope	Parsnips
Carrots, Sweet-	Peaches
Cauliflower	Pears
Celery	Pineapple
Chard Leaves	Potatoes, Sweet
Cherries, Sour	Potatoes, White
Chestnuts	Quinoa
Cucumbers	Radishes
Dates, Dried	Raspberries
Figs, Dried	Rutabagas
Grapefruit	Sauerkraut
	Soy Beans, Green
	Sea Vegetables
	Spinach, Raw
	Sprouts
	Strawberries
	Tangerines
	Tomatoes
	Watercress
	Watermelon

Registration for Monthly e-mail: "Better Breast Health Minute"

To register to receive our quarterly (or monthly) breast health note "Better Breast Health Minute" by e-mail, visit www.BetterBreastHealthforLife.com.

Websites

For your convenience, the websites listed in this book are available as hotlinks on the audio workshop CD. Just insert the CD into your computer CD driver and use your file directory software to open the Website document on the CD. Each website is listed in the order it appears in the following text. Just click on the website link of your choice to launch the website. (Requires an active Internet connection.)

1   How Does Breast Cancer Develop?

For more information on all known breast cancer types, their frequency of occurrence, treatment, and prognoses, visit the American Cancer Society website www.cancer.org/docroot/CRIcontentCRI_2_4_1X_What_is_breast_cancer_5.asp.

2   How is Breast Cancer Detected?

For more information on breast cancer detection and testing, visit the American Cancer Society website www.cancer.org/docroot/CRI/content CRI_2_4_3X_How_is_breast_cancer_diagnosed_5.asp?rnav=cri.

3   Genetic Factors

For more information on gene testing and the risk associated with these inherited genes, visit the National Cancer Institute website http://cis.nci.nih.gov/fact/3_62.htm.

To determine if your BMI correlates to a higher risk of adverse effects on health, determine your body height in feet and inches and your weight in pounds and then visit the National Cancer Institute website http://cis.nci.nih.gov/fact/3_70.htm.

4   Estrogenic Factors

For more information on the risks and benefits associated with menopausal hormone use, visit the National Cancer Institute website www.cancer.gov/clinicaltrials/digest-postmenopausal-hormone-use and the U.S. Food & Drug Administration website www.fda.gov/cder/drug/infopage/estrogens_progestins/default.htm.

To explore birth control methods, visit the U.S. Food & Drug Administration websites www.fda.gov/opacom/lowlit/brthcon.html and www.fda.gov/fdac/features/1997/babytabl.html.

5   Environmental Factors

For more information on endocrine disruptors visit the National Resources Defense Council website www.nrdc.org/health/effects/qendoc.asp#disruptor.

For a list of the top 40 potentially harmful ingredients commonly used in personal products, or to check the ingredients on the labels of your products, visit the website www.antiagingchoices.com/harmful_ingredients/toxic_ingredients.htm.

For purchase information on beverage bottles made exclusively of plastic materials not known to leach harmful substances, visit the Blender Bottle website www.blenderbottle.com.

For purchase information on polypropylene baby bottles made by Medela and their Day Carrier Kit , visit the Amazon website www.shopping.com/xFS?KW=Medela+ Accessories&FN=Baby+Care&FD=85708 or the Baby Mania website www.breastfeedingaccessories.com/cooler_ carriers.html.

For a list of known environmental pollutants and toxins from the Environmental Protection Agency, visit www.epa.gov/ebtpages/pollutants.html.

For a Citizen's Guide to Pest Control and Pesticide Safety, visit www.epa.gov/oppfead1/Publications/Cit_Guide/ citguide.pdf.

For the latest Report on Carcinogens from the Department of Health and Human Services, visit www.nih.gov/news/ pr/jan2005/niehs-31.htm.

For the Environmental Working Group's study on the toxic effect of various chemicals in our food supply, visit www.foodnews.org/effects.php.

For a list of environmental pollutants and toxins from the National Institutes of Health, visit http://ntp.niehs.nih.gov/ index.cfm?objectid=72016262-BDB7-CEBA- FA60E922B18C2540.

For more info on EMF, visit the National Cancer Institute website http://cis.nci.nih.gov/fact/3_46.htm.

6   Health & Lifestyle Factors

For more information on sunlight and vitamin D, visit the Oregon State University Linus Pauling Institute Micronutrient Information Center at http://lpi.oregonstate.edu/infocenter/vitamins/vitaminD/.

For more information on a Fit for The Cure event near you, contact a store near you or visit www.nordstrom.com.

For more info on the lymphatic system visit Wikipedia's on-line encyclopedia at http://en.wikipedia.org/wiki/Lymphatic_system.

Consult local authorities or www.epa.gov/waterscience/fish/states.htm for advisories on contaminated or polluted fishing areas and about the safety of fish from local lakes, rivers, and coastal areas.

For more information on mercury, consider visiting the Environmental Protection Agency, the Environmental Working Group, and the Audubon Society websites www.epa.gov, www.ewg.org, and www.audubon.org.

7   Dietary Factors

Visit the alkaline/acidic food charts at www.essense-of-life.com/info/foodchart.htm. You can also visit the on-line metabolic typing questionnaire at www.metabolictyping.com.

For more information on anti-cancer diets, visit Ask Dr. Sears at www.askdrsears.com/html/4/T040300.asp.

For more info on fiber, visit the Harvard School of Public Health at www.hsph.harvard.edu/nutritionsource/fiber.html.

For perspective and more information on the various forms of fats visit Ask Dr. Sears at www.askdrsears.com/html/4/T041300.asp, the Harvard School of Public Health at www.hsph.harvard.edu/nutritionsource/fats.html, and Women-to-Women at www.womentowomen.com/LIBcholesterolandfat.asp, and Udo Erasmus, author of *Fats that Heal Fats That Kill*, at http://www.udoerasmus.com/FAQ.htm#1_1.

To help identify which oils to use at various cooking temperatures, visit the Spectrum Organics charts at www.spectrumorganics.com/index.php?id=182.

For more information on glycemic index and load lists, visit the websites www.mendosa.com and www.glycemic index.com.

For more information on how cooking methods impact nutrients, visit the U.S. Department of Agriculture's Table of Nutrient Retention Factors, at www.nal.usda.gov/fnic/food comp/Data/.

For more information on the potential implications of microwaved foods on our health, visit the Global Healing Center at www.ghchealth.com/microwave-ovens-the-proven-dangers.html and www.buergerwelle.de/pdf/microwave_cooking.pdf.

8   Assessing the collective effect of all risk factors on breast health

For more information on thermobiological risk ratings and vascular display grades with thermal breast imaging examples **in color**, visit The Thermogram Center website www.thermogramcenter.com.

9   Lessons in Breast Care... Lessons for Life!

For information on Glenna's campaign and poster purchases, e-mail glennabiehler@msn.com.

For information on thermal breast imaging, visit www.thermogramcenter.com or e-mail info@thermogramcenter.com.

For information on self-exams, mammograms, and ultrasound, visit www.cancer.org.

Additional Websites & Organizations:

For more information on cancer and women's health, visit:

American Cancer Society: www.cancer.org

American Cancer Society Cancer Survivors Network: www.acscsn.org

BeeHive: www.thebeehive.org/health

Breast Cancer Action: www.bcaction.org

Breast Cancer.org: www.breastcancer.org

Breast Cancer Prevention Institute: www.bcpinstitute.org

Cancer Prevention Coalition: www.preventcancer.com

iVillage Health: www.ivillagehealth.com

MSNBC Health: www.msnbc.msn.com

National Alliance of Breast Cancer Organizations: www.nabco.org

National Breast Cancer Coalition: www.natlbcc.org

National Breast Cancer Foundation: http://nationalbreastcancer.org

National Cancer Institute: http://cis.nci.nih.gov/fact/4_18.htm

Susan G. Komen Foundation: www.komen.org

WomenCentral: http://womencentral.msn.com

Women's Information Network Against Breast Cancer: www.winabc.org

Y-Me: www.y-me.org

For more information on today's Thermal Imaging, visit:

Any of over 10,000 published research articles at MedLine:www.ncbi.nlm.nih.gov/PubMed/

A review/history of breast thermography studies: www.breastthermography.com/infrared_imaging_review.htm

For medical journal abstracts of numerous thermal imaging applications: www.thermology.com/research.htm

A Healthy Living article on The Thermogram Center: www.thermogramcenter.com/Images_files/Healthy%20Living.jpg

Protocols, training, and certification: www.iact-org.org For information on the importance of appropriate and qualified imaging centers: www.breastthermography.org/rogue.htm

Notes

[1] Smith R. et al. *American Cancer Society Guidelines for the Early Detection of Cancer, 2004.* CA Cancer J Clin 2004; 54:41-52.

[2] *Breast cancer: a reassuring look at the odds.* Health, January 1993.

[3] *Vital Signs.* Health, October 1992.

[4] Anderson D. *A genetic study of human breast cancer.* J Natl Cancer Inst 48:1029, 1972.

[5] Ottman R. *Practical guide for estimating risk for familial breast cancer.* Lancet 2:556, 1983.

[6] Love, S., Lindsey, K. *Dr. Susan Love's Breast Book,* 2000.

[7] Saltzen S.L. *The association of ethnicity and the evidence of mammary carcinoma in situ in women: 11,436 cases from the California Cancer Registry.* Cancer Detect Prev 21(4):361-9, 1997.

[8] Paskett E.D., et al. *Cancer screening behaviors of low-income women: the impact of race.* Women's Health 203-26, Fall-Winter; (3-4) 1997.

[9] *Breast cancer and body shape.* Annals of Internal Medicine 112:182-86, 1990.

[10] Petrelli JM, Calle EE, Rodriguez C, Thun MJ. *Body mass index, height, and postmenopausal breast cancer mortality in a prospective cohort of U.S. women.* Cancer Causes and Control 2002; 13(4):325–332.

[11] Hoy C., Stoddart. *The truth about breast cancer.* 1995.

[12] Kelly P. *Understanding breast cancer.* 1991.

[13] *Breast Cancer and pesticides.* Soil and Health January 1994.

[14] U.S. National Institutes of Health. *NCI HTML Cancer Bulletin for April 13, 2004*, vol. 1, no. 15.

[15] *Hormone Replacement Therapy and Breast Cancer Relapse.* Lancet February 7, 2004.

[16] Lanfranchi, A. and Brind, J. *Breast Cancer: Risks and Prevention.* Breast Cancer Prevention Institute; Aug. 2005.

[17] U.S. National Institutes of Health. *Oral Contraceptives and Cancer Risk.* NCI Cancer Facts 11/03/2003.

[18] *Pill ups cancer risk in young women.* Science News June 10, 1995.

[19] *Oral contraceptive use and breast cancer in breast cancer risk in young women.* Lancet 973-982; 1989.

[20] *New England Journal of Medicine* 328:176, 1993.

[21] Chris J. *Women who breastfeed.* American Health April, 1994.

[22] LaCecchia V.L. et al. *Reproductive factors and breast cancer: an overview.* Soz Praventivmed 34:101-107, 1989.

[23] *Broccoli inhibits cancer – mostly.* Science News 442, December 1994.

[24] *Ecocancers.* Science News 10-13; July 3, 1993.

[25] Lark, S. *21 day cancer miracle.* The Lark Letter, 2004.

[26] National Institute of Environmental Health Sciences. *Environmental Health Perspectives* Oct. 1993;101:372-7.

[27] Fackelmann K.A. *Breast cancer risk and DDT: no verdict yet.* Science News April 23, 1994.

[28] Weed S. *Breast Cancer? Breast Health!* 1996.

[29] Whelan E., *Menstruation and reproductive history study.* American Journal of Epidemiology December 15, 1994.

[30] Weil A. *Pollutants linked to breast cancer.* Natural Health November/December 1993.

[31] Redfearn, S. *fertile ground.* Natural Health September 2005.

[32] Rothschild-Levi, J. *Plastic Planet.* Delicious Living Feb 2005.

[33] National Institute of Environmental Health Sciences. *Environmental Health Perspectives* May 26, 2005.

34 Muñoz-de-Toro, M et al. *Perinatal Exposure to Bisphenol-A Alters Peripubertal Mammary Gland Development in Mice.* Endocrinology vol. 146, no. 9 4138-4147, 2005.

35 Knopper, M. *The perils of plastic: your cling wrap could be leaching chemicals - Your Health.* E: The Environmental Magazine Sept-Oct, 2003.

36 Whittelsey, F.C. *Hazards of Hydration.* Sierra Magazine.

37 www.breastcancer.org, Aug. 2005.

38 Sternglass and Gould. *Breast cancer: evidence for a relation to fission products in the diet.* Int. J. Health Services vol.3, no.4, 1993.

39 *Public testimony before Texas officials: breast cancer and radiation.* Feb. 22, 1994.

40 Stewart A. *Study shows risk in low-level radiation.* American Journal of Industrial Medicine March 1994.

41 Fackelmann K.A. *Do EMFs pose breast cancer risk?* Science News 388; June 18, 1994.

42 Keith L. et al. *Circadian rhythm chaos.* Int. J. Fert. 46(5):239-247, 2001.

43 *Cigarettes tied to fatal breast cancer* and *Fatal breast cancer and smoking.* Science News June 4. 1994.

44 *Alcohol and the breast.* Journal of the National Cancer Institute 85:692, 722, 1993.

45 *Letter* from Graham Colditz, M.D., Ph.D., Assoc. Prof. of Medicine, Harvard Med. School, published in Mother Jones, July/August 1994.

46 Hudson T. *Breast Cancer Prevention with Nutrition.* Women's Health Alternative Medicine Report 3-4; July/August 2000.

47 Holick MF. *Vitamin D deficiency: what a pain it is.* Mayo Clin Proc. 2003; 78(12): 1457-1459.

48 Northrup, C. *Women's Bodies Women's Wisdom,* 2002.

49 Grismaijer D. *Dressed to kill: the link between breast cancer and bras.* 1995.

[50] Thune, Inger, Brenn T., Lund E., Gaard M. *Physical activity and the risk of breast cancer.* New England Journal of Medicine 336(18):1269-1275, 1311; May 1, 1997.

[51] Jancin B. *Exercise study may point to hormones as the breast cancer culprit.* Family Practise News 5; Nov.1, 1994.

[52] Pelton, R. et al. *Drug-Induced Nutrient Depletion Handbook.* 1999-2000.

[53] Andrews, T. *The Healer's Manual,* 2002.

[54] Colbert D. *What you don't know may be killing you!* 2000.

[55] Crenson S. and Mendoza M. *Health officials look at mercury content in fish.* Daily Camera October 13, 2002.

[56] U.S. Food and Drug Administration/Environmental Protection Agency. *What You Need to Know About Mercury in Fish and Shellfish.* EPA-823-R-04-005, March 2004.

[57] Peat R. *Thyroid: misconceptions.* Townsend Letter for Doctors November 1993.

[58] *Journal of the National Cancer Institute* 87: 110; 1995.

[59] *Role of antioxidants in cancer prevention and treatment.* Townsend Letter for Doctors October 1993.

[60] Balch P. and Balch J. *Elements of Health.* Prescription for Nutritional Healing 2000.

[61] Gittleman, A. *Getting thin–on fats The healthy, sure-fire way with omega oils.* Eat Fat Lose Weight, 1999.

[62] JAMA June 2002.

[63] Chambers AF, Hill R. *Tumor progression and metastasis.*

[64] *Breast Imaging Study.* National Cancer Institute: breastimaging.cancer.gov/background.html August 27, 2004.

[65] Los M, Voest EE. *The potential role of antivascular therapy in the adjuvant and neoadjuvant treatment of cancer.* Semin Oncol 28:93-105, 2001.

[66] www.imaginis.com/glossary, Aug. 2005.

[67] www.thermascan.com/physicians.ivnu, Aug. 2005.

[68] Gautherie M. et al. *Accurate and Objective Evaluation of Breast Thermograms.* Thermal Assessment of Breast Health 1983.

[69] Gros, C., Gautherie, M.: *Breast Thermography and Cancer Risk Prediction.* Cancer 45:51-56, 1980.

[70] Louis, K., Walter., Gautherie, M.: *Long-Term Assessment of Breast Cancer Risk by Thermal Imaging.* Biomedical Thermology 279-301, 1982.

Index

Better Breast Health - for Life!™
ORDER FORM

Full Name ————————————————————————

Title or Mr./Ms./Mrs./etc. ————————————————————

Organization, if applicable ————————————————————

Shipping Address ——————————————————————

City/State/Zip ———————————————————————

Daytime phone ———————————————————————

Evening phone ———————————————————————

E-mail address ————————————————————————

PHONE	FAX	MAIL
For credit card purchases or more information call toll-free: 866-492-2174	Fax this 2-page form complete with credit card information to 303-664-1146	Mail this 2-page form with your check, payable to: BHEG P.O. Box 674 Louisville, CO 80027

All orders must be prepaid by check, Visa, or Master Card

For credit card purchases, check one ☐ Visa ☐ MasterCard

Cardholder's Name ——————————————————————

Credit Card Number ——————————————————————

Expiration Date ———————————————————————

Billing Address ———————————————————————

City/State/Zip ———————————————————————

See over →

Qty	Description	Unit Price	Total Price
	Better Breast Health - for Life!™ - 1-hr. Audio Workshop CD Guides listeners through the Risk Factors Worksheet, provided on the CD in Macintosh and Microsoft file formats. (The Actions Checklist Worksheet is also included on the CD.)	$3.95	
	Better Breast Health - for Life!™ - Book (includes above CD) Provides explanation and resources on the risk factors linked to breast cancer. This action-oriented book provides women simple, straightforward information on risk reduction strategies.	$18.95	
	Better Breast Health - for Life!™ - Risk Factors Worksheet Lists the risk factors linked to breast cancer and areas of opportunity to impact breast health. Used with the Audio Workshop CD, women can identify and prioritize the risk factors and areas of opportunity specific to their lives.	$1.00 for 10	
	Better Breast Health - for Life!™ - Actions Checklist Lists every risk-reducing action step included in the book in a checklist format so that women can identify, or "check", the actions they intend to take, and track their progress over time.	$1.00 for 10	
	Better Breast Health - for Life!™ - LIVE Workshop at your organization Led by Breast Health Education Group personnel, these interactive workshops lead women through their Risk Factors Worksheet, provides details and action-oriented information on risk reduction strategies, and culminates with completion of the Actions Checklist.	Call for details	

Shipping & Handling
(Orders are shipped via U.S. Postal Service)

Amount of Order	Add	Amount of Order	Add
Up to $20	$3.50	$60.01-$80.00	$8.00
$20.01-$40.00	$5.00	$80.01-$100.00	$9.50
$40.01-$60.00	$6.50	$100.01+ or priority/express mail: call for details	

Sales Tax: Colorado residents only: add 3%

Subtotal	
S&H	
Sales Tax	
Total	

Better Breast Health - for Life!™
ORDER FORM

Full Name _____

Title or Mr./Ms./Mrs./etc. _____

Organization, if applicable _____

Shipping Address _____

City/State/Zip _____

Daytime phone _____

Evening phone _____

E-mail address _____

PHONE	FAX	MAIL
For credit card purchases or more information call toll-free: 866-492-2174	Fax this 2-page form complete with credit card information to 303-664-1146	Mail this 2-page form with your check, payable to: BHEG P.O. Box 674 Louisville, CO 80027

All orders must be prepaid by check, Visa, or Master Card

For credit card purchases, check one ☐ Visa ☐ MasterCard

Cardholder's Name _____

Credit Card Number _____

Expiration Date _____

Billing Address _____

City/State/Zip _____

See over →

Qty	Description	Unit Price	Total Price
	Better Breast Health - for Life!™ - 1-hr. Audio Workshop CD Guides listeners through the Risk Factors Worksheet, provided on the CD in Macintosh and Microsoft file formats. (The Actions Checklist Worksheet is also included on the CD.)	$3.95	
	Better Breast Health - for Life!™ - Book (includes above CD) Provides explanation and resources on the risk factors linked to breast cancer. This action-oriented book provides women simple, straightforward information on risk reduction strategies.	$18.95	
	Better Breast Health - for Life!™ - Risk Factors Worksheet Lists the risk factors linked to breast cancer and areas of opportunity to impact breast health. Used with the Audio Workshop CD, women can identify and prioritize the risk factors and areas of opportunity specific to their lives.	$1.00 for 10	
	Better Breast Health - for Life!™ - Actions Checklist Lists every risk-reducing action step included in the book in a checklist format so that women can identify, or "check", the actions they intend to take, and track their progress over time.	$1.00 for 10	
	Better Breast Health - for Life!™ - LIVE Workshop at your organization Led by Breast Health Education Group personnel, these interactive workshops lead women through their Risk Factors Worksheet, provides details and action-oriented information on risk reduction strategies, and culminates with completion of the Actions Checklist.	Call for details	

Shipping & Handling
(Orders are shipped via U.S. Postal Service)

Amount of Order	Add	Amount of Order	Add
Up to $20	$3.50	$60.01-$80.00	$8.00
$20.01-$40.00	$5.00	$80.01-$100.00	$9.50
$40.01-$60.00	$6.50	$100.01+ or priority/express mail: call for details	

Sales Tax: Colorado residents only: add 3%

Subtotal	
S&H	
Sales Tax	
Total	

110